I'LL

MOVE

OVER

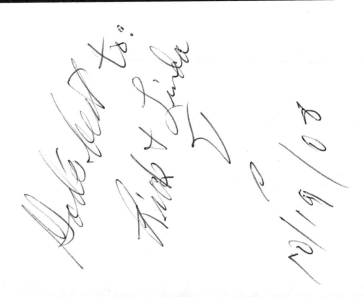

I'LL MOVE OVER

Spouse and Family Stress in
Dealing With Alzheimer's Disease

J. ROBERT BOGGS, JR.

With special contributions by

SCOTT R. PUCKETT
DARLENE ROHRER
CAROL J. VAN PELT
BARBARA JO McMUNN
AND
MARTHA L. SCHAFFER

Published By

J. Robert Boggs Jr.
1408 Camelot Dr.
Winona Lake, IN 46590-5602
(574) 372-6315

Contents

Contents

To:

DORIS MAXINE

Lifelong Sweetheart-Wife

for her

fierce loyalty

and

contagious, undying love

Acknowledgments

My first thought is "how can one person owe so much to so many?" Foremost, I gratefully acknowledge that I am happily and hopelessly indebt to God for life, health, joy and. . . .

Of the "many," I want to confess my indebtedness to two groups: family and friends.

My ten sisters and I had parents and grandparents of high moral/ethical/religious principles. Though we grew up in rural Georgia during the depression years with little cash, we were wealthy in the things that really matter. We used the words little, but **love** and **loyalty** we practiced with no pretense.

Hence, when "little brother" started to write a book, my sisters and their families joined our daughters and theirs to believe **that I could do it! And should!** My youngest sister, Martha, let me use a few of her excellent poems. Robbie, the next, and her husband, J.T., generously helped design and compose the first edition of the book via their computer.

My niece, Kathy Alley, was a great inspiration and Howard, her husband, graciously offered the art work.

James and John, husbands of our daughters, Carol and Barbara, gave help, love and encouragement. Carol wrote the excellent chapter on helping the family through caregiver stress, and Barbara allowed me to use two of her poems.

Now the circle really enlarges: Friends! Hey, folks, I gotta' quit! I can't write another book! **Thanks** to you **all**. "Poseyville" kin and friends; Bremen High School. My English teacher, Gladys Eubanks, and drama coach, Mrs. H.D. Hatchett.

Our Assistant Director of Nursing at Grace Village, Darlene Rohrer, did the "Inside Look" chapter. Scott R. Puckett, the C.E.O. at a great and beautiful retirement facility, Wesley Manor, in Frankfort, Indiana, did chapter ten on selecting a nursing facility. Maybe it's out there, but I have never seen anything that even comes close to the valuable, practical things he contributed. That one chapter greatly enhances the value of the book!

Edna Pringle helped more than she ever knew in her volunteer writing class in Warsaw! Dr. Donald Demaray – a patient teacher – prods, encourages and never gives up. Carole Streeter, sharp critic of writing, could have devastated but gently challenged instead. Dr. and Mrs. Otis Bowen gave a real lift when most needed. Dr. Mark Blaising and his wife, Nona, were most encouraging.

To these, a few of my family and friends, along with so many more, I hereby acknowledge with a grateful heart my great indebtedness.

– JRB

Introduction

How well I remember the day Rev. and Mrs. Boggs walked through the front doors of the nursing home. Their faces looked familiar, but I just couldn't remember where I had met them.

Arm in arm they walked up to the nurses station, and Mr. Boggs introduced his "Maxine" as our new resident. You could see the love in his eyes for her. But you could also feel hurt and a bit of hesitation in his voice at the prospect of entrusting her care to yet another group of strangers.

I asked him where they were from and he told me they had been serving as pastor and wife in churches of the North Indiana Conference of the United Methodists since 1952. I suddenly remembered that it was at pastors meetings and youth camps I had seen them several years back.

As we walked Maxine to her room, she clung silently to her husband's arm. In her room, we began showing them how to operate the bed and the call light. Mr. Boggs interrupted: "But my Maxie won't remember to use the call light."

How my heart ached for him as I remembered taking my own mentally retarded son to a home for handicapped children. I felt that no one could possibly love him or care for him like I could. But I also knew it was a 24-hour job.

In my heart I wanted to try to let Mr. Boggs know that we would do our very best to care for his Sweetheart wife and keep her safe. I assured him that we have a "nurse alert" cord that we pin to her clothing, so that if she became restless and tried to get up, it would pull the call light on and staff would come to assist her.

As time passed, we have shared what Maxine could still do for herself and the things she liked to do; like playing the piano, reading and walking. Playing the piano and reading both faded out after about a year. Two years later she quit trying to talk. But for three and one-half years she is still able to eat well and take two walks each day with her husband.

From the inside, some of us get a pretty clear picture of the broad spectrum of people and their family life and backgrounds. As time has passed, our staff have come to admire Mr. Boggs' devotion to his wife. With all the broken marriages in our society around us, the Boggs have been a real inspiration to all of us. Even though Maxine does not speak any more, you can see her love returned in a smile or the tender kiss she always has for her husband when he comes to her. If you could have been here with the approximately 300 people to help them celebrate their 50th wedding anniversary on July 10, you would have been deeply touched as he sang to her "I Love You Truly."

— DARLENE ROHRER, Grace Village
Assistant Director of Nursing

Before You Begin

The author has spent time and effort to make this book as helpful as possible to the growing multitude among us who wrestle with a big problem: Alzheimer's disease or related dementia. The subject at hand is neither religion nor theology, though a personal faith is reflected without apology, especially in chapter six.

Government agencies, church and community organizations plus many great-hearted individuals have contributed to our family's survival of the Alzheimer's crisis. There is **hope** and **help** out there for each of you who may be staggering under a similar load. We've survived – and with **joy** – and we believe **you** can, too! I always enjoyed stories with a happy ending. That's the way I expect our story to end. It is our fervet hope and prayer that you "live happily ever after," too.

Thanks for sharing your time and heart with our family and the millions of other victims who are now in the throes of a literal life-and-death struggle with a slow but nonetheless deadly **killer**.

– J. Robert Boggs

"SOMETHING'S WRONG WITH MY HEAD"

Recognizing Symptoms

IT WAS DECEMBER 20, 1987, at a rest home in Warsaw, Indiana. Our stroll in the halls was over. My wife, Maxine, was tucked into bed at 9:00 p.m.

"Let me kiss you good night, Sweetheart. It's time for me to head over to my little apartment."

"Oh, please don't leave me, Honey! You don't have to go back to Grace Village tonight. Just stay here with me." To her it sounded so reasonable; so simple and easy.

"How I wish we **could** stay together, Sweetheart!" I assured her. "But I doubt if your roommate would approve."

"Oh, it would be OK with you, wouldn't it, Mabel? Mabel was silent. (Which does not always "give consent.")

"But Sweetheart, even if Mabel didn't mind, the nurse would come in shortly and boot me out."

"Oh, no she wouldn't! She wouldn't mind at all. Honey, **please!** – just stay right here with me tonight!"

With my heart doing strange things inside me, I took a deep breath and said slowly: "Sweetheart, even if Mabel did not mind, nor the nurse object, I still couldn't stay here. Where would I sleep?"

"Right here with me."

Looking from her beautiful, pleading eyes to the single hospital bed, I replied:

"I'm afraid there isn't enough room on that one little bed for the two of us."

"Oh, sure there is! **I'LL MOVE OVER!**"

What a spirit! What an attitude! So ready to "adjust" with no thought of any inconvenience to herself. With Alzheimer's disease (AD) slowly destroying her brain, the reasoning was faulty, but what a **heart** of **love**! No wonder I fell in love with such a beautiful person years ago in our college days!

Without wavering, she has shown that attitude all these years during joys, bereavements, and still more joys. (Joys. I mention twice and bereavements once. Two-thirds vote is a good, strong majority in any election!)

Some people think they can't win for losing. It seems to me that we can't lose for winning! I hope you can catch a little of that spirit and attitude in *I'll Move Over*!

*   *   *

The earliest I can recall even the possibility of anything being amiss in Maxine's mental health was about 20 years ago when she was 51. Occasionally, she would put her hands to her head and say, "Bob, there's something the matter with my head."

"You mean you have a headache?" I would ask.

"Well, no. Not exactly. But my head doesn't feel right." For my needed enlightenment, I would question from every angle. Finally, she would say, "I can't explain to you just how I feel. But one thing I know: my 'thinker' doesn't work like it once did."

What was I to say to that? My usual reply was, "I suspect your brain is getting rusty. Maybe you should use it more." Most of us tend to say insensitive things like that when we don't know what to say, don't we? (St. Peter had that same problem. See St. Mark 9:5-6, *NIV*.)

For the next ten years we happily pursued our occupation and calling, and rearing the last two of our four children. Occasional comments about her head persisted.

Neither we nor very many other people in those days had even heard the term "Alzheimer's disease." But in retrospect, I recognize that symptoms of AD began to appear. Memory loss seems to be one of the most prominent in the list of most people, but many other little things came along with it.

For clarity, let me share with you a quote from Dr. Peter Davies' *Alzheimer's: An Overview*, p. 6. Aronson et al).

"The symptoms of AD include gradual declines in:
• memory, learning, attention, and judgment;
• disorientation in time and space;
• word finding and communication difficulties, and
• changes in personality.

These symptoms may be somewhat vague at first and mimic mental illness or stress-related problems . . ."

I hope you will take note of that list of symptoms for future reference. The list is not exhaustive, but it can serve as a foundation on which to build understanding of AD.

*   *   *

A quote from a paper I found that our daughter Barbara wrote for a college class might shed some light on those years following my first vague recognition that something unusual might be going on.

"The next stage in Mom's life went unnoticed for several years. In my time at home as 'one of the Boggs girls,' I don't remember many Sunday dinners alone as a family. Mom expanded many a 'six-mouth' meal into dinner for ten or twelve. She did this on a very humble budget, enjoying every minute of it. Her love for God and for people shone through these impromptu, simple, but nutritious meals, served so often to unexpected guests, friends or transients.

"After my sister Betty's death, Mom began showing preliminary signs of AD. Like a noticeable memory loss, excessive worrying and unnecessary anxiety over very ordinary occurrences. At this point none of us knew what was affecting her personality, but through it all she taught me (and us) the true meaning of fortitude. Her faith in God never wavered. She always believed that God was in control of all things, including her life. She kept busy, directing her energies toward:
- loving and serving God, who was first in her life;
- graciously caring for her husband and family, and
- finding ways to helpfully serve and love other people.

Then in the summer of 1984, Mom began to forget how to prepare food properly. Dad had to be close by to answer her repetitious questions. This is when my father determined there must be something wrong and took her to a doctor."

*   *   *

Looking back, most of us who have a family member with Alzheimer's disease can point to a time much earlier than we first identified as the beginning of symptoms.

"Hindsight is always 20/20" we often say. The statement is not literally true, but it has a big grain of truth in it.

Although each case is unique, there is a broad base of symptoms common to almost all Alzheimer's patients. If you are dealing with Alzheimer's disease or related dementia (ADRD) at this point in your life, we hope you will find helpful information and inspiration in the retracing of some of our family's trek across this wilderness.

In retrospect, most of us can remember things that signalled the fact that "something was working on" our loved one for quite some time. We charitably dismissed it with "all of us are getting a little older" or "as we grow older we all tend to develop a few peculiarities."

In my wife Maxine's case, she was really not getting all that old yet. She was only 52 when at least one friend later said he had noticed a difference in her. Usually, we don't think of people in their early 50's as being candidates for ADRD.

My first thought was that perhaps the emotional stress of losing our only son in a car accident when he was 19, followed by the death of her mother (to whom she was very close) just five months later, was responsible for changes I thought I was seeing in Maxine. Before recovering from these losses, her father died.

Still ahead lay a very rugged and uncharted road: the shock of again facing that ruthless intruder called cancer. This time to snatch away our oldest dauthter, Betty. (To which our daughter, Barbara, alluded.)

Musically talented, bright, with a sparkling and outgoing personality. That was our Betty. She was also a dedicated Christian, happily and effectively serving God as a pastor's wife. She and her husband, Jerry Kissinger, had an adorable two-year-old son, David. Then entered little and cute Ruth Ann.

Five weeks later, April 1, 1974, our Betty had a massive lung hemorrhage and died in fifteen minutes. It was an awful **mauling** for us all but especially for Maxine.

All of which made me wonder if there might be a connection between great emotional trauma and ADRD. I'm confident those on the scientific investigative end of it have thought of that angle already. Especially since research has concluded long ago that stress in general has a decided negative effect on many diseases, and our health in general.

October, 1984 – Alzheimer's begins to "close in"

Coming home in the evenings, I would check the pad by the telephone for calls I was to answer. Increasingly there were incomplete numbers with no name by them. "Sweetheart, was I supposed to call someone?"

"Oh, yes! Someone called and wanted you to call them when you got home! I don't remember who it was, but the number is there by the telephone." It's frustrating to find part of a telephone number and no name with it.

It's also a shock to come home for a meal and find a strong odor of a "burnt offering" that was earlier intended to be your dinner. Or to find enough food prepared to feed a big family with only the two of you there to eat it! Another shock is to be about half way through a big meal and smell meat burning in the oven – when you already have meat on the table.

Along with memory loss came difficulty in making quick decisions, like responding to "turn right at this corner."

Frustrated, she would ask: "Which way is right?" That would often strike my "funny bone."

"You mean you don't know the difference between your right and left hand?"

"Of course I do, Silly. It's just that I grew up in Kansas where we always directed with "north, south, east or west." That sounded reasonable at the moment, but later I could see that it was a subtle **coverup** for the inability to make quick decisions.

No one likes to be singled out as "having a problem." Especially when that problem only hinders our normal function perhaps 2 percent to 5 percent of the time.

"Well, you forget things too, don't you?" she would say.

"Yes, Darling, I do. But I'm thankful that, for now at least, I don't forget as much as you do!"

Can you see why a basic sense of good humor helps so much in the small daily stresses of life? Many of you could say with me: "I have God and laughter to thank for the measure of sanity and normalcy that I enjoy."

When young people began to say, "Wow! Maxine is some driver!" I began to wonder. She had always been a safe, polite, conservative driver.

"Did she scare you? Did you have a close call?"

They would reply, "Well, she did pretty well, but we did have one or two 'close calls' on the way."

It is fairly normal in city driving for any of us to have a "close call" occasionally. But if they get too frequent, it might be reason to look for other symptoms. Especially if the diminishing skills are accompanied by a tendency to get **lost** in **familiar territory!**

Most, if not all of us, have been telling a story and lost our train of thought right in the middle of it. Embarrassing, isn't it? But if the *occasional* becomes **frequent**, it's a whole new story. It may be time for medical consultation. Not from panic, but concern. Maxine's loss of memory had now reached that point.

I took her first to our family physician, who referred us to a neurologist. After a brief preliminary examination at the office, it was off to the hospital for an EEG – and all the other initials you're all familiar with – to try to get to the bottom of the great memory loss she was experiencing. (My thought was that perhaps the blood flow to the brain was becoming inadequate to keep it functioning well.)

Finally, all tests finished, we looked across the desk at the doctor who held the papers with the printout of our earthly destiny. He first gave Maxine a few simple memory tests. Like, "Who was our last President?" She failed it. Then he said, "I'll give you a simple four-word sentence that I want you to remember and repeat to me in a few minutes. Say after me: 'The purple fox ran'." She repeated it, and I was confident she could remember so vivid a sentence. After a few minutes he asked her to repeat it.

"Well, I think it was something about a fox." But she was not able to repeat the four words. (I remember them vividly nine years later!) Shuffling the papers again, he looked up at us and said:

"You passed all the tests at the hospital with flying colors. Physically, you're in perfect condition for a 62-year-old. But your loss of memory and the total overview of your case leads us to the conclusion that you have what is called Alzheimer's disease."

In concert, we both asked: **"What is that?"**

Then the good doctor carefully explained to us that the German psychiatrist and neuropathologist, Dr. Alois Alzheimer, had done research on patients with brain disorders and had discovered by autopsy two unusual things: neuritic plaque made up of degenerating nerve terminals and a fibrous material called amyloid. The second abnormality was neurofibrillary tangles. (The word **tangles** we understood!)

Then the doctor tried to get it down to our level: "For all practical purposes, the brain of the AD patient dies, just a few million cells each day. Since the human brain has billions of cells, it usually dies slowly. Sometimes very slowly. And the brain actually shrinks in the process."

Then he shared a very prophetic word – one that we saw no need of at the time: "You indicate that you have never heard of the disease. Many people haven't heard of it, but you will certainly hear more about it in the future. Cases of it are getting more numerous all along. You will probably want to get acquainted with other families affected by it and join a **'support group'** to share your experiences and insights."

Every word the doctor said was right on target. He outlined the progress and stages of the disease, saying that each individual case moved at its own pace, but always ended the same. And with no cure yet in sight.

He was also right in predicting that we would need to join a **support group**. Only 18 short months later our AD "survival kit" included regular group sharing in a support group.

At this juncture the stable predictability of life for Maxine and me suddenly took wings. One thing I did know: Our mutual promise to keep each other "in sickness and in health" had top priority with me. I felt about Maxine exactly like Dr. Robertson McQuilkin said he felt about his wife Muriel when she began to suffer from Alzheimer's. He resigned as president of Columbia Bible College to take care of her. In his chapel resignation speech, he said:

"In a way, this decision was made 42 years ago when I promised to care for Muriel 'in sickness and in health till death do us part.' As a man of my word, integrity has something to do with it.

"But so does fairness. Muriel has cared for me fully and sacrificially all these years. If I cared for her the next 40 years, I would not be out of debt. Duty, however, can be grim and stoic.

"There is more: I love Muriel. She is a delight to me – her child-like dependence and confidence in me, her warm love, flashes of that wit I used to relish so; her happy spirit and her tough resilience in the face of her distressing frustration. I do not **have** to care for her. **I get to!**"

Signs of Trouble

When memory loss begins to affect a person's life, it's a problem. Most people in the early stages of the disease belittle the problem or pass it off as "getting old." In fact, many people retain their memories very well as they age, having as good or as bad a memory as they ever had.

The disease progresses like this:
• fading memory;
• personality changes;
• trouble with talking and moving;
• difficulty concentrating;
• problems with routine activities like combing hair;
• poor judgment (dressing for winter in July);
• confusion and disorientation;
• loss of bladder and bowel control (person may also forget how to find the bathroom);
• can't recognize loved ones or friends, and finally,
• loses awareness of where he/she is, what day it is or who's around him/her.

Few people suffering from Alzheimer's die from the disease itself. Most die from pneumonia. Life expectancy for Alzheimer's victims is cut by 30%.

Recognize

Symptoms

With

Patience

and

Love

THE NATION'S "MOST DEMOCRATIC" DISEASE

Who Are These ADRD Victims?

WITH OUR AGE-SPAN constantly climbing, we now have more than 4.4 million Americans with some form of dementia. One-third of that number must have help to do the simple, every-day things like eating, dressing and toileting.

Who are these victims of Alzheimer's disease? College professors, rocket scientists, top business executives, factory workers, housewives, and any other walk of life, educational or social strata you care to name. Someone said that AD is the "most democratic" disease among us. You may have caught that just from watching TV specials about it.

It seems to many of us that AIDS gets a lot more press and attention than cancer and ADRD combined. AIDS is a dreadful disease. All reverent and caring people pray and hope for progress and help toward its early solution. We must not lessen our concern about it. It is **critical**. We must get to the **root cause(s)** with all dispatch and **honesty**. Desperation about it may lead us to the discovery/admission that AIDS is as much a moral problem as a medical one. The real truth is, while funding is important, **you can't solve a problem just by throwing millions of dollars at it!** True science follows wherever truth leads. Our search must have honesty as a light on the path. And a bit of humility would do us a lot of good, too. Let us seek to become true scientists and we'll get farther faster.

But let us not forget that cancer and ADRD are also pressing medical and financial problems in our society. Actually, the two combined are a much bigger problem than AIDS. Perhaps not as serious, but much larger at the present.

There are some fifty conditions that can cause dementia. Among people 65 and older with dementia, AD at least contributes to the condition of 70% of them. Strokes account for 20%. That leaves only about 10% for all the other dementia combined. That indicates the prominence of AD among us in this country.

Let me share a quote from Peter Davies, Ph.D., from a book I consider one of the best, most authentic and definitive works on the technical aspects of ADRD I have seen. It is called *Understanding Alzheimer's Disease.* – What It Is – How to Cope With It – Future Directions. (An excellent gathering of medical and writing talent, edited by Dr. Miriam Aronson, of New York. See Ref.)

"AD and related dementia pose a threat not only to those who are afflicted but to their families, friends, and ultimately to our society. The threat is so great that AD has been called 'the disease of the century' by Lewis Thomas, noted physician and author. Former Health and Human Services Secretary Margaret Heckler said in a 1984 report: 'When we find a cure for AD, we – as a people – will release and reap a now untapped harvest of wisdom, insight, and experience from millions of Americans in their golden years.' (Aronson et al., p. 4.)

"Persons eighty-five and older represent the fastest-growing age group in our population. Those over seventy-five are most vulnerable to AD. By the year 2000, the '75+' group will make up at least one-half the number of those 65 and over."

Please note: Although more than one-half of those showing signs of dementia will actually have AD, many of the others will have conditions that are treatable. That is why I am suggesting that if you or a family member begin to show these signs in an uncharacteristic or noticeable way, a talk with your physician would be a good idea.

Let's review symptoms:
- a marked, though gradual, decline in memory, learning ability, attention span or judgment;
- disorientation in time and space – getting lost in a familiar area;
- frequent groping for words – communication difficulties;
- changes in personality. (Aronson, et al, p. 6.)

Many of the above I have noticed in my wife, Maxine, for the past nineteen years.

As AD began to tighten its grip on her brain in 1984, she was heroic in resisting it, but it was a losing battle. Although somewhat relieved to know I had not been secretly "imagining things" for ten years, the agony and trauma of our situation was excruciating. Retirement plans had to be accelerated by at least two years. Our plans to winter in Florida, except for the first year after our retirement, had to be scrapped. You can see why such turmoil often sends caregivers into real depression.

When I was tempted to feel sorry for myself, I would muse: "Lord, I'm not the one needing sympathy. After all, it's my sweetheart wife who has the disease!" Thus, I found help to keep the focus of my attention, love and prayers for **her** rather than on myself, which was much better.

My "Maxie" put up a valiant fight. She had known for ten years that "something" had a strong hold on her brain. When she found out what to call it, she seemed not to have the slightest thought of "giving up" or giving in to it.

Once or twice she had some difficulty loving a couple people who did some thoughtless and rude things. This was unusual for her. Talking with her and praying together at these times was enough to pull her through with no "big deal" made about it. (It was usually she who helped **me** through many a rough spot!)

Hopefully you're getting the idea that the "marvelously and wonderfully made" human brain is just as vulnerable to malfunction and disease as any other part of the body. It is no disgrace to have a bad heart, diseased kidney, or pancreas. No stigma is attached to any of these. Please tell me then: When will we mature enough to think of the brain as just another important part of us? A body part that often has malfunctions that are treatable and often curable?

I hope you're also getting the idea that many of your acquaintances, friends, neighbors and yes, perhaps some members of your own family may be one of the many millions who already are victims of ADRD. Often a dementia has been at work on its victim for five or ten years before it can be detected. We are all alike in two things: We think it's the sort of thing that happens to "other people." We're also united in the fervent wish that if some part of our body does get sick, it will not be our brain.

Victims of ADRD are scattered throughout the population indiscriminately, and they are in all stages of development of the disease.

You will **not** find these ADRD victims nor the "victim families" out demonstrating, screaming, or threatening politicians if they don't give us what we want or think we need. But we, with quiet reason, appeal to the sense of fairness of our fellow-Americans: Please don't forget us. Let your hearts be big enough to include us in the re-doubling of efforts in research and concern. Remember: The brain you help rescue and preserve could be your own!

Caregivers Are Also Victims

Sixty percent of nursing home residents have some kind of dementia. Their care costs billions of dollars annually. But what you may **not** know is that **most** of the more than 4.4 million dementia patients in our country are cared for **by family members at home.** And each of these family members are **secondary victims** of the illness.

We all owe a debt of deep gratitude to the faithful **caregivers at home** who without fanfare and often without much thanks, care for a family member. Many of us are simply not equipped emotionally or financially to do it.

Real heroism touches us deeply. These caregivers are heroic in the finest and best sense of the term. Just remember: For every hero whose statue stands in a park some place, there are thousands of living heroes who stand in the shadows. They have not won the world's applause by their faithfulness in caring for husband, wife, child or aged parent. (Nor have those who faithfully go to work every day to make an honest living and pay taxes.) But heroes they are.

Applause, ability and visibility do not comprise the standard by which we humans ought to be judged or rewarded. I believe that **faithfulness** is one of the BIG words. It is a word with which our generation needs to get re-acquainted. Let us all be encouraged to believe that it is an attainable standard for each of us. (See *Moody Bible Inst.,* Ref.)

The extremely intricate computers called "brains" in 4.4 million of us are ill. Multiply that number by the number of family members **indirectly** affected by ADRD. Now you are just beginning to get a picture of the staggering number of us called its "victims."

No wonder Dr. Lewis Thomas has called AD "the disease of the century!" Almost every family in America has someone in the family or extended family with ADRD! We need to awaken to this fact, and to an awareness of the billions of dollars we must spend annually in the compassionate care of the victims. Financially, we **all** are victims of ADRD! But why not view this as a challenge and opportunity for real progress in mental health and brain disease?

One of the first big steps forward could be a change of attitude. Again, why should a disease of the **brain** carry a stigma that a disease of the **heart** does not? Think now of all the ribald jokes the mentally ill have had to endure for centuries! That fact alone reveals a deep sickness in our human nature. We need to find a cure for the "sick" attitude we humans have toward mental illness. Learn a sad history lesson from Hitler and Nazi Germany! Either we learn from the mistakes of history or we are bound to repeat them. Hitler used the mentally ill for "scientific" causes.

Who are these ADRD victims? We ALL are victims! Just remember, the brain you help save may be **your own.**

Those of us considered "normal" tend to forget that we could be one of the victims of ADRD some day. Our life-span gets longer at a steady pace, and with it an increasing percent of us will be victims. Since dying younger is the alternative, most of us want to live and take our chances.

If that unhoped-for illness should be your lot one day, how would **you** want to be treated? Herded along with other unfortunate souls to be used as a human "guinea pig" for experimentation in scientific research projects like Hitler did? Any "volunteers"? No. We would each like to be treated with dignity, respect and compassion, whatever our age or condition.

There is good reason why the Golden Rule really is **"Golden."**

"In everything, do to others what you would have them do to you, for this sums up the law and the Prophets." (Matthew 7:12, *NIV.*)

ALZHEIMER'S DISEASE
WHAT IT IS – WHAT IT IS NOT

Alzheimer's Disease *is:*

- A progressive, dementing, fatal brain disease
- The fourth leading cause of adult deaths in the United States
- The cause of more than 100,000 deaths annally
- A "democratic" disease – found in every segment of the population
- An emotional and financial nightmare for victims and their families
- An economic time bomb for the decades ahead

Alzheimer's Disease is *not:*

- A natural part of aging
- A mental illness
- Easily diagnosed
- Covered by government or most private health insurance
- Limited to the elderly
- Curable

3

WHAT CAN WE DO TO HELP?

Supporting Cast

WHEN FORCES beyond your control thrust you into the fast lane of life's "discipline of the difficult," you will need help. No need to kid yourself or spend valuable time wishing. Just accept the fact that your smooth road has suddenly turned rocky. To survive the Alzheimer's "wilderness trek," you will need:
- at least two good doctors and a good working relationship with your available medical community;
- a caring and faithful family;
- a vital faith and a caring religious fellowship;
- an ADRD support group, and
- government/community agencies.

No attempt was made to list these in the order of their importance. That varies with each of us, but our family has been fortunate to have the big plus of a real lift in each of these areas.

Yes, we all forget at times. Yes, any of us may become temporarily disoriented on occasion. No, **my** logic need not always make sense to **you**. But with these problems **accentuated** (and a few other things thrown in with them for a family member), it is natural to turn to your GP or family doctor for help. If he thinks the situation should only be watched a while, he will say so. If he thinks the symptoms warrant, he will refer you to a neurologist who specializes in diseases of the brain and nervous system.

Your next stop may well be a hospital or clinic for a check to see if there are other things causing the symptoms.

"There are two points to be kept in mind. One, the majority of elderly persons who exhibit symptoms of dementia will turn out to have AD. Two, there are other causes of dementia symptoms that may be treatable. Thus, every person with these symptoms deserves a thorough medical investigation." (Dr. Peter Davies, 1988, p. 5, *Understanding Alzheimer's . . .*)

Again, Dr. Davies says (p. 7), "A diagnosis of AD can be considered when other causes of dementia have been ruled out and the findings are consistent with AD. This diagnosis can be **confirmed** (emphasis mine) only by brain biopsy or autopsy." For practical reasons, understandably, that confirmation of diagnosis most of us never bother about. All we need is a reasonable prognosis with which to work.

You are fortunate if you have a physician not only skilled in science to give you the concise and adequate information you need, but who is also kind, sympathetic and human as he breaks the news that you hate to hear.

Blessed Are the Caring Families

Having grown up in a large, caring family and having had four very devoted children leaves me unable to sympathize with those of you who are not so fortunate. But I am keenly aware of the value of the heritage with which Maxine and I have been blessed, and am deeply grateful. In no way do I feel worthy of such true wealth, but at least I am thankful. I can also try to express that appreciation by being "surrogate family" to the several I've found in need of same. Many have family, but they live too far away to be of much practical help. Moral support can be carried on at a distance, and is not to be discounted, but we often need hands-on help.

About eight years ago when Maxine and I needed help and comfort the most, our daughters and their husbands organized to take turns coming to visit us on Saturdays. This they did for more than a year at our most crucial time. What a lift! And what memories our whole family has to enrich the rest of our lives. Their children were taught lessons of love and family loyalty they can never forget.

What Can We Do to Help?

It was October when the crisis of AD broke upon our heads. But even our "accelerated" retirement could not take place until the following June 1. What could I do? How could I make it, with Maxine's memory slipping so fast?

She loved people and enjoyed making calls with me, so I began to take her with me wherever it seemed appropriate. She loved our people and they freely returned her outgoing love. Some did not even guess she was wrestling with AD for quite a while.

With all the pastoral responsibilities and the concerns at home, one can understand how my rising level of anxiety might start to show. Our church people began to wonder what they could do to help.

Pretty soon one of the leaders of a women's group said to me: "Pastor, we know you have calls to make and studying to do. We are organizing among ourselves to take turns taking Maxine shopping two mornings a week and keeping her out for lunch. That way you will have at least two days a week with large blocks of time to do whatever you need to do."

God bless the women! Talk about "angels of mercy!" For us, they began to flutter down from heaven – in human form – and without wings!

"If We Can Just Make It to June 1!"

By the time of our big retirement banquet the folowing June, the "teacher" had been taught a lot about caring for his fellow humans. How could one ever forget people like that? It was a **long** eight months, but **together** we made it to June 1!

A vital faith in a living, loving God was a giant factor in it. A "community of faith" with practical, down-to-earth, caring people helped more than they will ever know. An excellent medical community helped to give us accurate, concise information to guide us concerning the future. We arrived safely at retirement. Whee!

*   *   *

Our "dream home" we had been slowly building in the lake country of northeast Indiana was just about ready to move into when we retired. We were

two hours from each of our two daughters, who faithfully came to visit us. It was my set purpose to take
care of my sweetheart-wife and try to do a little long-
delayed writing. After a short while, I saw that the
caregiving took about 24 hours a day and the writing
was put on the shelf.

Support Group – So Helpful!

It did not take very many weeks to discover what
the good doctor meant. "You'll probably find yourself
wanting to join a **support group** of other people
with a problem like yours." He was right on target!

The closest group we found was in Ft. Wayne. It
was about forty miles each way, but well worth the
drive.

A support group usually consists of eight to 14
people. This one met at the State School for the
Mentally Handicapped. Many groups meet in hospi-
tals. We met once a month with one big purpose: to
share experiences and information on how we were
making it. Several of the patients came with their
caregivers (usually a spouse, but sometimes another
family member). They were usually not as vocal in
the participation as their caregivers, which is under-
standable. But the fact that many were present is
indicative of the "open-ness" of the meetings.

Often a medical doctor or social worker would
come and make a presentation of information that
we always were eager to hear. Doctors were very
helpful with updates on the latest discoveries/-ex-
perimentations with the disease. Those informative
talks kept us in touch with efforts to help solve
our problem on a long-term basis. But it seems as I look
back that the greatest benefit was the sense of belong-

ing, fellowship, and the flow of ideas from all the other caregivers who were actively wrestling with the same struggles we had. Twelve people can come up with a lot more ways to solve a problem than one or two can.

After several months of traveling 40 miles to Ft. Wayne, Maxine and I discovered there were about eight or 10 other families right in our own county with Alzheimer's. It did not take us long to help organize our own support group there. The local hospital gave us a place to meet. Doctors and nurses freely gave of their time to meet with us, speak to the group, and be helpful in every possible way.

Services for Families/Caregivers

There are many helpful community and governmental agencies available to the victims of ADRD and their families. The number and nature of services varies with location and the size of the communty. Your needs may not be the same as someone you know. And your needs do not stay the same as the disease progresses!

What kind of available services? Health and mental health agencies. Private practitioners. Crisis teams.

Then there are the socialization/nutrition places, with their senior centers, congregate meals, Meals On Wheels, friendly visiting/buddy systems, etc.

The Office On Aging proves helpful to many, with information, referral and advisement. Then there are our governmental "entitlement" programs. There is Medicare, Medicaid, veterans' benefits/Social Security disability benefits.

One of the most helpful programs we found was the Respite Care services. We used the adult day care a few times, which was not real expensive and very helpful. But the Respite Care program we valued the most was the one where once a week a "relief person" came for four hours to give respite to the caregiver.

For a caregiver to be able to depend on a four-hour time-slot to go shopping, fishing, visiting or ? every week proved to be a great help. I don't know what it costs our government, but think of the millions of dollars it saves in postponing the necessity for institutional care! Add to that the value of the improved mental and physical health of that great army of home caregivers, and you begin to see the true worth of this Respite Care program.

Our nation spends billions to take care of people in nursing care facilities. But the bill would be more than twice as much if it were not for the great number of people who take care of family members at home. The amount we spend aiding these caregivers and helping to keep them mentally and physically healthy is one of our best investments.

We all need each other. Neighbors need each other. If you want to be a high risk for a crackup or a breakdown, just hold tenaciously to the notion that you can single-handedly lick any problem that comes your way. That attitude will help assure that you will "self-destruct" sooner or later.

Don't Be "Silly" – Be Smart As A Goose!

Betty Malz, author of the best seller, *My Glimpse of Eternity,* has some interesting things to share about geese. She insists they've had a **bad rap**. They are not "silly" as often called, and have much to teach **us**. For instance, they have a good reason to fly in a "V" pattern. The "top goose" or "head honker" is an experienced navigator. He knows the terrain and the way to where they want to go. And the "honking" you hear is not just noise. It has meaning and purpose. They are encouraging their leader. He has to crash through the wind resistance for the rest of the group. In the "V" pattern, the wings of the first goose creates an air lift for the one behind him. With this pattern they can **all** fly seventy-one percent farther than they could by flying "solo"!

When the leader gets tired, he drops to the back where the flyng is easiest. Then one of the "lieutenants" takes the lead. They learn to share the load of leadership. If one goes down ill (or for any reason), one or two others go down with him to help him while the main flock moves on. They plan to aid each other in recovery and join the flock farther on.

Incidentally, geese are monogamous. (Strange, when I typed that word on my spell-right word processor, I got a "beep." I spelled it every possible way and still got a "beep." Then I looked it up in my big old two-volume dictionary and found that I was right in the first place! Apparently the word **monogamous** is omitted from a modern word processor! A "sign of the times" maybe? Oh, I know. It was just one of those "freak" omissions. Maybe.)

Who is "silly"? Geese? Or is it people who think they can "go it alone"? We really do all **need each other**. We can't make it alone. Survivors learn that they need God and other people; family, friends, and community. Nations may finally learn that they also need each other. Wouldn't it be great if the fear, greed and hate in us were replaced with the spirit of trust, caring, and helpfulness?

*   *   *

Although the **caregiver** may seem to be the "hero" in the pre-institutional care of AD, I hope that I have made it clear that without a "**supporting cast**," no individual could last very long. To close this brief but vital chapter, let me share with you excerpts; one from an AD patient and one from a caregiver, from the Duke Family Support Program publication *The Caregiver* (Spring, 1993, Vol. 13, No. 1).

'I regret and resent bitterly the lack of human touch. Always a very physical person, now I find people pulling away as though my hand were rotting flesh. Alzheimer's is not contagious. It is not violent, although I admit to an inner boiling rage at circumstances. . . .' 'I wish my neurotransmitters would permit my understanding of this "neuroglitch from hell" and why it affects others as adversely as it affects me. . . .' 'I cannot come to terms with being neutered. . . . No longer a woman, just an empty vessel who still enjoys the touch of luxurious fabric . . . and a stroking hand.' (See *Living in the Labyrinth* by Diana Friel McGowin under "Helpful New Resources," p. 13.)

Try to Remember . . . by Bill Wiley, a caregiver. "When I became a caregiver, I knew absolutely nothing. . . . Like most caregivers, I had to learn everything from the beginning. . . . Most of us were thrust into the role . . . Eventually we read, we question, we attend meetings and workshops and we begin to learn. . . . Caregiving is never easy, but the job is easier if we can remember a few important truths:

Remember, these people did not choose to have this devastating and eventually fatal disease. . . .

Remember, our loved ones often experience anxiety, loneliness, confusion and the feeling of being lost in time and space. Anything we do to comfort will benefit them and us.

Remember . . . , no amount of coaxing, scolding or nagging will replace what is missing. Those particular brain cells are gone and will not return.

Remember, the ability to reason or think logically decreases with age as the disease progresses. Arguing will not help. Admonishing will not help, and the use of logic will definitely not help.

Remember, affection and acceptance **will** help your loved one and you, both now and when this affliction has run its course. (Courtesy of the *Honolulu Chapter Newsletter.*

Yes, for **inter-dependence**, we were designed and made. The sooner we learn it, and act like it, the better.

ADJUSTING TO
EARLY INVOLUNTARY RETIREMENT

Learning to Live With ADRD

WE HAD SLOWLY BUILT our own "dream house" for retirement. It was almost finished when we had to move in – two years earlier than we had planned.

I became the caregiver for Maxine, which meant that I did, or closely supervised, the cooking, laundry, housework, yard work and whatever else needed to be done. I was "on duty" 24 hours a day, seven days a week, except when we were both asleep. I knew nothing about **caregiving**, especially the "around the clock" kind. I had to learn, and fast. And I'm still learning.

For almost forty-two years of married life, Maxine and I had been real "sweethearts." With love like ours, I never considered my role a burden, but a privilege and a joy – as I know she would have done for me had the roles been reversed. I approached the task with zest, even though it was certainly not like the retirement we had once planned.

We were soon introduced to the government's **Respite Care** program, taking advantage of the weekly four-hour respite given by the visiting caregiver. It was a great help. Our monthly **AD Support Group** was also a real boost to our morale, teaching us more and more of what we needed to know about how to cope with Alzheimer's disease.

What a lift our two daughters and their families brought by their bi-weekly Saturday visits! (One small problem. They are both excellent cooks. The food they brought made my cooking after they left look "sick" by comparison!)

At times Maxine would take a look at what I had prepared for dinner and say, "My stomach doesn't call for that right now."

My usual reply was, "Just tell your stomach to 'get with it' and eat what I've prepared. I know I'm no great chef, but it's good, nutritious food. Besides, I worked really hard getting this stuff ready!"

After reluctantly nibbling at the food for quite a long time, she would come out with a bright, sweet smile and enthusiastically say: "You know what my stomach calls for right now? Some good ole' ice cream!" Our bantering usually ended with hearty laughter, and my giving in to let her dive into the ice cream, after just a few more bites of the meat and veggies I had prepared! (I dutifully drove a hard bargain.)

Incidentally, if you lose that sense of humor, you're a "dead duck" in the swirling tides life, and especially in times of crisis.

Except for two months in Florida the first winter after retirement, and occasional trips to visit family and friends, we lived the next two years in our little "castle" nestled in the lake region of northeast Indiana near Angola.

The sudden change from being 63 with "full employment" to the isolation of retirement living might have been even more traumatic had it not been for the small church a few miles southeast that needed a "preacher" on Sundays. I'm not sure we did Alvarado Church a lot of good, but they helpfully served as a "bridge" for us at that crucial time in our lives. Sudden retirement can leave one with a feeling of isolation. For **that** feeling (and condition), the Creator did not make us.

*   *   *

Around a conference table at a corporation meeting a member of the board – perhaps the chairperson – says: "Let me bounce this idea off your backboard and give me your reaction." So the group squares off to trade shots of logic.

"As iron sharpens iron, so one man sharpens another" is the way Proverbs 27:17 puts it. The idea and the need is as old as the human race itself.

Families do this all the time. All of us know that if a young child has siblings, he/she can be expected to learn to talk at a younger age. Adult members of a family bounce ideas off each other regularly, to their mutual benefit. We live by logic more than we realize.

Downsize Your Logic for ADRD Patients

We say: "It's a crazy world we live in!" Perhaps. But the world and our society is more reasonable than the statement implies. Those who take seriously adjusting to life with an AD family member make that discovery. When shooting a rifle, adjustment must be made for wind velocity, or you'll miss your target. So must we make adjustments in our logic when dealing with an ADRD patient. They still operate by logic also; not yours, but one "tailor-made" for their exact condition at that precise moment in their lives.

We adults often smile at a child's conclusions, and seldom hesitate to point out to them where they're "wrong." We try to give them pointers in coming to a more "mature" position. If a precocious child wants no part of our adult reasoning, we even override, overpower or "pull rank" on them. This may cause resentment in the child, but that risk must be weighed against the possible bodily harm if we **don't** restrain them at times.

But what if the faulty judgment in question is by an adult? And what **if** you cannot convince them to change their minds by argument, reason, or any sophistry that comes to mind? Restraining them may pose a much greater problem than you would have with **any** normal child!

No "One Size Fits All" Answers

Learning to live with someone with a dementia is not as simple and easy as some might suppose. But it can be done. (With a lot of adjusting.) More than two million valiant Americans are doing it now for a loved one. Most of them for love, not money, just because they care.

Their first thought when hit with the problem likely was the same reaction you would have: to **run**

away. Have you ever noticed that our first reaction to a problem is almost always the wrong response? These **caregivers** thought it over. Many will tell you they prayed for wisdom. They concluded that trying to run from a problem was no solution at all, but a quick way to get into more and **worse** difficulty. (Just as many are now concluding who have thought about divorce.) So they stayed and sought for real answers. Asking for wisdom at every turn, they received it. (James 1:5)

*   *   *

You may still be saying: "OK, I believe all that. But **how** can we learn to adjust and live helpfully with a family member with ADRD?"

My first word to you is: (a) decide and determine to remain **a caring person**, no matter what. That involves emotions, but even more it is an act of the **will**, and (b) learn to **think**. And to out-think your patient. If you don't, you will get bogged down emotionally. A friend of mine loved to say, "Use your head, Bob! God expects you to. Otherwise He might as well have put feet on both ends!"

In the Appendix, please look for the rather long list of "Do's and Don'ts" garnered from the wide experience of many people. Workable, practical things. Some from institutional caregivers and some from personal experiences at home. I hope you will review it, and add your own discoveries to the list.

If an unusual loss of memory is the first noticeable sign of AD, I would put next a **subtle** loss in judgment, or ability to reason properly. Let me give a few "for instances."

Where's the Fly Swatter?

When most of us see a fly in the house (especially if it is on the table), our reaction is "Where's the fly swatter?" That was always Maxine's reaction until AD began to tighten its grip and her power to reason began to suffer.

"Oh, no! Don't kill the poor little thing! It has a right to live. Why not catch it and put it outside?"

Have you ever tried to catch a fly or ant to depose them to the out-of-doors?

"You've got to be kidding!" would be the usual prelude to the execution of the insect, be it fly or ant.

But she was quite serious. After out-voting her a few times (which, fortunately, she soon forgot) and carrying out the death sentence on insects, it occurred to me that the loving girl I had married years ago was still that same compassionate person I had the privilege of living with now! And **what a discovery!** More valuable than any hidden treasure I've ever heard about.

It was only a part of her brain that was dying, fouling up her usual ability to sort things out properly. When I finally saw her in that true light, I came to a love for her that far surpassed any sexual attraction I had ever had (and that was **great**). And the magnetism of her personality now drew me to her more strongly than her beautiful, innocent smile had once been able to draw me straight to her from across the room or across the college campus back when it was beautiful young love!!

Behold, I kid you not! It is because of this glorious discovery more than six years ago that I now labor to put a small bit of this **reality** into printed words in hope that many others may come to know this **far greater love**.

I am trying to tell you about this quality or dimension of married love that far surpasses the glory and beauty of sexual love. Even the pure, conjugal, relationship of a husband and wife who have known only each other, and for many wonderful years, as glorious as that is.

When you find **"a glory,"** you have discovered something too wonderful to describe, almost too good to believe, and yet too grand not to attempt to share.

Like the teacher in Alaska who found her art student admiring a beautiful sunset. When the teacher suggested that she try to put the scene on canvas, she replied: "Oh, I can't draw glory."

Men and women who blend their spirits and bodies in pure and holy sexual love as God planned and intended find such a **glory** that the thought of even trying to describe it seems not only futile but a defiling sacrilege.

Then I should not be too surprised if some of you look at me askance when I tell you there is a dimension of marital love that is yet **more glorious** – that we're enjoying and have been walking together in – for six years now.

Too good to be true? No, too good **not** to be true! I know many of you will find it hard to believe, even though you would like to believe it. Those of you who have discovered the reality of this love, perhaps long before I did, are yelling **"Yes!"** deep in your grateful hearts! When you are party to a reality this wonderful, it makes you want to **shout it from the house top**, or from the highest available mountain! Just writing about it puts me "far up" somewhere.

It's hard to come down from this mountaintop, but you may be asking: "Did you then stop swatting flies and killing ants to adjust to Maxine's new way of looking at insects?" Well, no. But I tried to swat the fly or squash the ant in her absence, Think! And you'll find that there is often more than one way to get the same job done. Caregivers of ADRD patients have discovered that often a problem will disappear if you ignore it, or refuse to make a "big deal" of it.

*   *   *

Once when I was helping with dishes I dropped one of our lovely plates. We both felt bad about it, but Maxine had a bright hope. "Don't worry, just gather up the pieces and you can glue them back together."

Again, she was serious. I have repaired broken plates, but not when one is broken into "smithereens." Having honestly expressed my doubts, I quietly swept up the pieces, and put them in a paper bag, supposedly to do the repair job at my convenience. Later in the day I placed the bag of parts in the trash bin for the garbage pick-up. Wouldn't you know it! Before the pick-up, Maxine found not only the bag of broken parts, but several other pieces of ordinary junk she began to return from the curb to the house.

How would **you** handle a situation like that? I don't think I did very well with it that day because part of it I have forgotten. But I do remember rather playfully throwing tin cans at each other and accidentally hit her on the head with one when she ducked, which she failed to appreciate or see any humor in. After our fun was over, there were tin cans and trash scattered about on the front lawn, all of which we both then had to pick up, piece by piece. It was not, as I remember it, one of my "better days" of diplomacy, but we got through it to better and brighter times.

Shoe Shopping

One day Maxine said to me, "Bob, look at these shoes! They're coming apart. I need a new pair."

"You are so right, Sweetheart! Why didn't you tell me sooner? We'll run over to Angola and buy you some shoes this very day." Finding shoes that fit and ones she likes was always a problem, but we finally found the answer at the JC Penny store near the old city square.

"We'll take this pair," I said. But before the sales-girl could wrap them up, Maxine interrupted with a question.

"How much are they?"

"They happen to be on sale today," she answered happily. "They're only $24.95."

Maxine looked shocked. "Twenty-four ninety-five! I've never paid that much for a pair of shoes in my life! Just forget it." (Her memory of prices had really done a "Rip Van Winkle"!)

Recovering from my shock, with Maxine looking at shoes on another rack, I whispered to the lady: "Alzheimer's. Put the shoes away and I'll come back for them later today." I returned later, alone, and bought two pairs, which Maxine wore proudly for many months.

Oversized Pebbles

My Sweetheart and I enjoyed strolling down the gravel road the two blocks to the main road to get the mail in the afternoon. Sounds sweet and romantic, doesn't it? It was, well, that is **after** I was willing to "adjust" to one of her new little habits that developed.

She started this strange thing of picking up little stones from the gravel road and carrying them in her hands. Any stone that looked larger than usual, she picked up. "What are you planning to do with those?" I finally asked.

"I'll take them home and put them somewhere in a safe place. I'm afraid they will hurt people's tires."

So that was the reason for this developing habit of stone collecting! Being such a caring person, she wanted to make the road for us and others as smooth as possible!

"Ah, come on, Honey! Let's go! Those large pebbles will not hurt car tires. People drive on gravel roads all the time. Don't you remember when we drove on nothing *but* gravel roads?"

She didn't remember, hence many a time I would have to help her deposit her collection of those "hurtful" little stones in a "safe" place before we went into the house when we returned from our "little date." I never changed her.

How would you handle a situation like that? Scold, and keep trying to reason with her? Continue a futile effort to get her to change her mind?

Why not *commend* her for being such a caring person? Why not make a "game" of it? You can smile or chuckle (in your mind) even while holding a straight face outwardly. Learn to **bend** a little! It won't *break* you. If you have a sense of humor, why not put it to work? It can save real distress for you and the one for whom you're caring.

Each issue that arises must be dealt with on it's own merit. Just realize that the patient is operating with a logic, even though it is not yours. Weigh issues and consequences involved as they arise. What is "true" or "real" to your patient may not be with you. We must learn to **step over to where they are** if we're to get along with them in a caring, ministering relationship.

May I share with you what I decided to do with the "collection" of little stones? Call me "Mr. Sentimental." But I still like the idea. I got a piece of velvet on which to arrange the stones in the shape of a winding path leading past a little rock garden. Some of you would be more artistic and creative, but to me the little path and tiny rock garden is enough. Know what I chose for the title at the bottom of the frame? *Because She Cared So Much!*

I know; we Irish are sentimental. Most of us will be ready to plead guilty to the charge. But the Irish are also loving, loyal people. You may wonder if I can look at my little picture without a tear or two. So what? Eventually, I figure the tear will be replaced with just a quick, loving thought of the vivacious girl with reddish-blond hair and a most winsome smile that I married fifty years ago. She has been a great lover, and I like to tell her that every day. How I marvel at the kind providence of the One who led me to her.

Resentments Into Love?

"Possibility thinking" you may call it. But it really is possible, with some creativity, to turn resentments and stressful situations into little symbols of love and appreciation. I dare you to try it!

Some people don't allow themselves to love deeply or completely because they are afraid they'll "get hurt."

How sad! And what an egotistical "excuse." Talk about hurting yourself! The most "deprived" people on God's earth are those deprived of love. and to think that most of the time we do it to ourselves, by not being willing to become vulnerable enough to love.

Some people have asked, "How will you take it when your Maxine is gone?" I don't know, but I have no intention of trying to cross that bridge before I get there. Having lost our only son to a car accident when he was 19 and our oldest daughter to cancer when she was 28, Maxine and I have experienced loss of the most agonizing sort. We have also happily had what you'd call "miracles," too. Like the two times years ago when Maxine was almost "done in" by cancer. (Carcinoma.) The first time she was only 28. The second time she was 56. By God's great "miracles," she came through both encounters to enjoy robust physical health – until AD sidelined her at age 62. Someone said, "There are a lot of things that will just have to wait for Resurrection Day." That pretty well sums it up. Meanwhile, we enjoy every mercy we find coming our way and learn to say, "Thank You" often and from the heart.

"Early to Bed and . . ."

Really, I don't know how to empathize with people afflicted with insomnia, because I have been blessed with the coveted ability to "lay aside my troubles with my trousers" and go to sleep shortly after I get comfortable and still. One little disappointment my dear wife had with me was for that very thing. In bed, she enjoyed quietly talking over the events of the day in review and plan for the next. I did, too, for about three minutes, and then I was "out" like a light. It really is annoying to be talking with someone and after a long pause there is no answer except deep peaceful breathing! But since she really loved me, she reluctantly learned to accept me as I was. (You just can't get *everything* in one, so why ask for the impossible?)

When AD caught up with her, it was I who had a problem. By 10:00 p.m., I was "beat" and ready for sleep.

"OK, Sweetheart, it's been a long day and I'm so tired. Let's 'hit the sack.' Is that all right with you?"

"Yes," she would reply. "I'm almost ready. Let me dry and put away these few dishes and I'll be right with you. I'm tired, too. You go on to bed and get it warmed up for us. OK?" That sounded like a cozy idea.

About 1:30 a.m., some unusual little noise must have awakened me. Seeing that her side of the bed had not been disturbed and that the kitchen light was still on, I got out of bed and stumbled into the kitchen. There she was at the sink, washing, drying, and putting away dishes.

"Sweetheart, you're gonna' wear those dishes out washing and drying them! Why didn't you come on to bed like you promised?" (The number of damp towels told me how many times she had washed, dried and put away the dishes.)

So went our early-morning conversations. It did not take long for me to realize that it was not safe to go to sleep while someone with a very decimated memory bank had the run of the place. I could think of dozens of possibilities that could be bad, or even disastrous.

For one thing, I imagined some "undesired" person coming to the door and her letting them in. Then I thought of the possibility that she might decide to take a walk.

"I'll fix both those problems," I said to myself. So I

decided to put locks on the doors that required a key to get in or out. It then occurred to me that we could not get out very fast in case of a fire. Finally, I elected to install small latches on the door high and low in the hope that she would forget how to open the door. That seemed to be most practical, and least expenseve, and it worked. This is part of what it means when we say: "You need to **Alzheimer's-proof your house**" when a loved one needs it for safety.

Learning by experience that getting my "Maxie" to bed when I went still had an occasional problem: her "clock" did not always call for sleep when mine did! Putting a child to bed may have its problems, but an adult? Having tried every alternative your tired brain presents may lead you to spank a child and let them cry themselves to sleep. But try that on an adult and you will feel utterly stupid! How about a sleeping medication? That helped, but since neither of us had been taking any medications, we still didn't like the groggy feeling during the day.

Please don't get the idea that I had – or found – all the answers. "Weak and human" describes me, too. At times my frustration was so great I actually said: "Hey, Kid, I'm trying to take care of you. If you don't learn to cooperate better, you're gonna' 'kill me off' and then who will take care of you?"

How cruel! Remarks like that would only add to her already high level of anxiety. She was doing her best already. In my frustration, I was asking her to do what she could not do, with a steadily dying memory. With flashes of clear insight and understanding, she would humbly apologize. Then I would humbly apologize to her. With "all forgiven and forgotten" and resting in each others' arms, we both would resolve to do better.

Sometimes "dropping" a worn-out, touchy topic did not last very long, but the five minutes was **bliss**!

The Lost Is Found . . . By Two Angels!

It was past mail time. I was busy, and Maxine wanted to walk the two blocks to the main road for the mail. "Why not, Dear? The walk will do you good."

When it was time for her return, I saw no sign of her. Soon I decided I'd better amble down the road to see who she had engaged in friendly conversation. Seeing not a soul, I began to knock on doors. Nobody had seen her.

Finally, I found one lady who said she had stopped at her house on the way **to** the mail box, but had not seen her since. With fear creeping toward my throat, I began to walk all the little streets and lanes of the neighborhood, enlisting the help of everyone. I was ready to go down to the lake (two blocks the other direction) or to call the sheriff's department. Looking at the sun as it lowered so fast in the west, fear began to tighten my abdominal muscles. I oped to call the sheriff. But before I could get into the house to call, an old pickup came chugging up to our house with Maxine and two older men I did not recognize.

The men said they had seen her several blocks west and sensing that she might be lost, they thought they'd best just bring her home. Said they had seen her around this house before, and figured she lived here.

Wheeee! What a relief! This time, God's angels came along *in overalls* driving an old pickup! You can bet I did not let her go even two blocks alone again.

Which Life Is Worth Saving?

Hitler decided that for the glory of the Third Reich

and the progress of the Aryan "Super Race," all babies born with any deformity should be destroyed. He also determined that retarded and mentally ill persons could best be used for medical experimentation. This would further science and help rid the tax rolls of "nonproductive" people at the same time. The marvel to all sane historians is that he was able to "sell" this idea to enough people in a country as highly developed morally and intellectually as Germany! But he "pulled it off" for the whole world to see. It shook our confidence in "the goodness of humankind" so thoroughly that it, hopefully, will never be quite the same again.

Working in the yard, Maxine got a small cut just below the knee. I cleaned it, put a bandaid on it and forgot about it. About a week later, she complained that she could hardly walk. Investigating, I found a swollen knee. Fast, I took her to the doctor, and he quickly had her admitted to the hospital with severe blood poisoning.

All the following week a great medical team fought to save her limb and her life. She couldn't figure out why she was there, or the reason for all the IV's, needles, and bandages. But we family members sat many an hour to help see to it that she didn't pull them out. She made it, and the life of one who was a "cripple" in two respects was saved. To us, her family, the life they saved was precious and very much worth saving. Tell me, who was right? Hitler or the Boggs family? Our family already decided. America is now in process of deciding issues just that weighty.

On the many trips I've been privileged to visit Israel, one of the most haunting and stirring things I see is the Holocaust Museum. The phrase that grabs my soul there is the words: **"NEVER AGAIN!"**

Brave words. But knowing human nature as we are beginning to, we need to admit that it not only can, but will happen again unless . . . (I was going to finish that sentence, but decided it might be better to let each of you finish it for yourself, which we actually must do anyway.)

Broken Things

At an interstate highway rest stop some time ago I saw Maxine taking something from one of the big trash cans. Moving over toward her, I interrupted her: "Sweetheart, put it back! It may have bad ole' germs on it."

Later, in the car, I noticed she had something in her hand, and asked if I might see it. Surrendering to me the "treasure" she had found, she said: "Let's take it home and repair it. You can fix it. I know you can!"

It was only a cheap "cracker jack" type of toy that a child had broken and carelessly tossed away. Hardly worth having when new. Now it was broken.

While I was thinking about how to diplomatically get it deposited in the car's litter bag, I had a strange and wonderful experience. With my sister driving us down the highway, it seemed for a little while that I was suspended somehow in time and space. And it seemed that I was suddenly seeing **people** and **things** from a higher vantage point. I saw broken people with crushed spirits; people who were valued by almost no one – except God.

I'm really a down-to-earth fellow who is not given to "visions" very often. And that one faded all too soon. I guess that's the reason I've remembered it so vividly all these years. But it left me with a question I'll share with you:

Do you know any "broken" people? If so, it might pay you to get near them. You may be surprised Who you find close by. (Psalm 51:17 and 34:17-18.)

5

VOICES CRYING
"TAKE HER HOME! TAKE..."

Adusting to Institutional Care

I F YOUR FAMILY is hit broadside by ADRD, **adjustment** will be "the order of the day" for some time to come. Then, just when you think everything is "under control" with care at home being provided by a spouse or other family member, the **caregiver** begins to show signs of physical/mental fatigue and a serious round of **re-adjustments** beginThat's the story of life, really. Adjustments and re-adjustments. There is within us a yearning for stability and continuity. That craving must be denied.

The ultimate change for each of us is death, which most of us want to dodge/postpone at all costs as long as we can. But there are many lesser changes before then.

When circumstances dictate – or strongly suggest – that the time is near to institutionalize a family mem-

ber with ADRD, here are a few of the adjustments that
you will face:

- loneliness;
- the family budget;
- daily schedule;
- recreational and social activities, and
- travel plans.

Looks as though with this starting list, one's whole
life will presently be re-arranged. Let's talk about
some of these.

Loneliness hits hardest the one who is institu-
tionalized. Though they may be surrounded by many
people, a feeling of isolation is still one of their big-
gest problems. Ask any one of them in any place
where they want to go and about 99% will say, "I
want to go home." Being in a crowd who are not
close family can leave one feeling like a lone wolf on
a vast prairie with no other ears to hear your howl.

The words "home" and "mother" probably top any
list of words with nostalgic potency. Picture this one
little 80-year-old lady pushing another one (near the
same age) around in a wheelchair. "I'm her mother,"
she explained. The one seemed to enjoy the free
ride, but even more, I think she liked being "moth-
ered," and once again being a daughter of her long-
lost mother. True, it was only a small part of a
family, but it seemed to help them both, for a while.

These days it seems to be sort of "illegal" to se-
date patients more than necessary, and I agree with
the idea, even though it causes another pretty big
problem. You have to put alarms on the doors and
electronic devices on quite a number of patients who
would rather walk out and go "home."

But patients are not the only ones plagued by

loneliness. Many **spouses suffer** also from the same, and some even more, since they must live alone.

Many widowed or divorced people have talked and written concerning the social difficulties of trying to find their place in a "couple oriented" society. The challenge is very real. Those who have mates in nursing homes feel the same isolation at times.

A sense of **guilt** must often be dealt with also. No matter how hard one has tried, still the lingering question may remain: Could I have done better or hung on longer? Remember, a sense of guilt does not have to be reasonable, logical or real to bother you. If the truth were known, it might be that more people suffer from false guilt than real.

Perhaps we ought to turn the question around and ask: "What might have happened had I **not** stepped from under the load in time? Two casualties rather than one?"

When to institutionalize is a big question. Since the caregiver is closest to the situation and is doing the work, she/he should have the "largest block of voting stock." Said caregiver knows more than anyone else how he/she feels. But there are times when family/ friends can detect signs that it ought to be done, even before the caregiver is willing to admit it. If you are considered a "patient" person and yet find your "fuse" getting shorter and shorter for no real good reason, it may be a "red flag." Take a look at it.

In our case, our daughters kept check on me regularly, and I felt free to tell them how I was feeling. Thus, it was a joint decision. That is best, if possible. But do not wait too long!

After we had decided that June 1, 1987, was to be "C-Day" – the day my dear wife Maxine was to be committed to the care of a nursing home (or perhaps "crying day" would be more accurate), a close friend of mine encouraged me by relating a sad story. His dad tried **too long** to care for his mother at home. One night during a north Indiana winter blizzard, she wandered out of the house. When he missed her, he called the county sheriff's department to help search. They found her body the next day in a cornfield not far from the house. "Bob, I think you made the right decision." It was a sad comfort, but a confirmation, nevertheless, that we had made the correct determination.

Budget adjustments have to be faced also. If you have been a hard-working, independent, pay-as-you-go person and have a comfortable "nest egg" saved for retirement, you may be in for a little shock. With the average annual cost of health care facilities at around $36,000 and climbing, your retirement "nest egg" may be spent in a few years. Even if you had $200,000 saved, it could disappear in about five years.

What can you do then? What most people have to do: Pay a visit to the local Medicaid office in your county and apply for help. This is no sure-cure tonic for a drooping ego, but one thing it can do: give you a feeling of kinship with the great mass of "common people" out there. That feeling may be humbling, but it is not all bad.

In that case, who pays for the rather expensive care? We all do. If you have worked and paid taxes, you will have **pre-paid** part of it yourself. Immediate family members who have sufficient income may be asked to share in the expense. The balance? Taxpayers in general. And, really now, most of us would much rather work and pay taxes to help care for unfortunate victims any day than to **be one** ourselves!

Victim families needing aid are allowed to own a car for transportation and a house or apartment in which to live, plus cash or liquid assets of about $2,250. Which means that if a family is asking taxpayers for help with a real need, it is only fair that they do what they can first and then share the financial load as they are able afterwards.

Your **schedule** is another thing you will need to adjust. Nursing homes are eager to have family come to visit. It helps them keep their patients happier, and if they are content it makes their work much easier. You will soon learn the visiting hours schedule and when meals are served. If there are special diet problems, you will tell them, and they will expect you to cooperate when you bring in little "extra" foods for treats.

The Administrator soon discovered that I now lived alone and that I came every day to visit. He informed me that for a small fee, I was welcome to come in at noon and have lunch with Maxine, which I happily did. On July 10, I mentioned to someone that it was our 44th wedding anniversary. When the Supervisor found out, she invited us over to eat with the staff personnel that day. They all began to tell what a great lady my Maxine was; how sweet, kind, helpful and thoughtful, etc. They had been sedating her to curtail her activity, so she just listened for a while. During a lull in the conversation, Maxine said with an uncharacteristic drawl:

"Well, you – know – what – makes – me – that – way, don't you? It's Jesus!" Suddenly a perfect silence fell over the whole group! Then, with a laughter of delight I answered:

"Yes, Sweetheart! Jesus in the heart makes a wonderful difference in the life!"

Often since that day I have thought: how **powerful** that **brief witness** was she gave to her faith! Many longer ones I've heard, but none any sweeter or more vibrant.

Recreational and social activities must be adjusted to fit with your new situation. At first, your friends may invite you to go along on a few special or selected outings, but increasingly you will find yourself moving in a fairly small circle (except for your family). Again, our society really is "couples oriented." You must deal with it.

Travel plans will never be quite the same, if you and your spouse enjoyed traveling together as Maxine and I did. My trips have been reduced to a couple days or at most 2-3 weeks. And going places is never the same when you leave half of yourself behind. One thing for sure: It is always a great delight to get home again!

Speaking of "home," I have noticed the past two days as residents of Los Angeles talk to TV news people about the earthquake of January 17, 1994, destruction of their **homes** seems to occupy "front stage center" in their concerns.

If and when my Sweetheart should not be here to come "home" **to**, it will be another difficult adjustment. I know.

Another adjustment a family must make is seeing your loved one in a place and situation you hope and pray that you will never be – without letting it depress you. Your family member will eagerly look forward to your visits, be they short or long. (Shorter ones, done more often, are preferred if possible.) If you are depressed when you come to visit, your potential to lift their spirits is greatly lessened. The people I feel the most sorry for are those who have no family to drop by with a cheerful little visit. By contrast, I see the "lift" for the ones who have family members or friends coming every few days (and some every day). With **delight**, I have noticed that several patients with no living family are fortunate to have friends to come regularly and cheerfully as surrogate "family."

I have heard people say: "I went to see Sally once after her stroke, and it depressed me. I don't intend to go again until her funeral. I want to remember her like she was during all those good years when we were close friends."

I have a thing or two to say about that utterly self-centered attitude: I hope and pray that God has given me a few friends of better quality than that, just in case I should ever be confined in a similar situation! How about you? I know a little about the value of the faithful love of **family** and **friends**. To me they are priceless!

What Is A Hug?

The bumper stickers that say, "Have you hugged your kid today?" proclaims a great need, documented by behavioral scientists. And it's not just kids who need hugs of affirmation. We all do! We may outgrow our need of much milk, but we never get beyond the need for the message sent by hugs. That assurance says: "I care about you." It is very simple and basic. Being held close, even briefly, conveys tidings of caring that every family needs.

I never knew, nor did our family know, *how*

valuable the simple, yet profound, messages conveyed so lovingly by Maxine's hugs. That is, until AD suddenly destroyed the "hugger connectors" in her brain. Let me explain.

July, 1987, Angola, Indiana

The family had gathered on that Saturday to see "Mom" at the nursing home. She had been there a month, and they had finally found the right level of sedation so that she was neither like a "zombie" nor running around trying to help any who requested it. We all had a delightful visit.

This "ordinary" day was made very memorable by those last, long and tender hugs for which my "Sweetheart" wife had long been known by those close to her.

With our daughter Barbara's permission, I want to share with you the poetic way she summed it up two years later. You'll learn something about Alzheimer's disease and feel part of the stress and grief process going on in one family as we **moved over** in adjusting to the crisis of AD, breaking up housekeeping and accepting institutional care of one greatly loved.

Yes, we miss those hugs. The six years have only deepened the longing to be "held tight" again by someone with such a powerful love to share. But we've adjusted, and together we're surviving.

THE HUG OF A LIFETIME

It began as many other visits –
    Sweetness mixed with loneliness;
Quietness mingled with discontent;
    Voices crying out from deep within:
      Take her home! Take her home!

It's never easy seeing Mom strapped to a chair,
    Or tied in a bed;
Her eyes reach out in much the same way
    That light stretches –
Into darkness.
    Never wanting to let go;
Wrapping around your heart and tearing at it,
    As you know you must go.

A mother's embrace!
    How special can it be?
I never really knew
    Until I had received my last one.

I recall vividly each embrace she gave that day;
    First, my sister, Carol;
My nieces, my husband, son and daughter;
    Then it was my turn –
For what I thought would be an old familiar
      good-bye hug:
    Something expected; something taken for granted.

But as my precious mother raised her arms,
    I knew something was different – very different.
Mother's embrace was l-o-n-g and tender
    As it had been with each one before me.

It was so full of love and expression –
    Beyond measure.
As I looked into her face,
    Jesus whispered to my heart
That **that** embrace would be my **last**
       from Mom this side of Heaven;
    And it was.

I cried then – as I am crying now,
    But what a Blessing and Joy
To look toward Heaven,
    With one more reason to love God
With all my heart,
    And live only for Him!

Heaven seems so far –
    So distant at times;
But Jesus says,
    "No, my child; Heaven is close – even within you."

Heaven! No night there! All sadness gone!
    No good-bye's!
Heaven! Only peace and rest;
    And **love**!
Heaven! What joys will be ours
    To embrace once again!

– BARBARA JO MCMUNN

HEAVEN'S HELP
IN SURVIVING STRESS

God's Inner Healing and Help

FROM OUR RETIREMENT on June 1, 1985, to the summer of 1987 my wife Maxine and I were **hurting**. She was struggling with the sure knowledge that she was "losing her mind." (The last thing any of us would want to lose, is it not?)

Caught in the vicious grasp of a merciless robber intent upon taking your memory, bit by bit, would you be frustrated/resentful? It is no wonder many AD patients have drastic personality changes. What member of their families would hesitate to admit that living with them is not quite as much "fun" as it once was?

The spouse and family are also victims of AD, whether they like it or not. The involuntary "election" to a difficult (and at times a seemingly impossible) assignment brings with it a pressing invitation to self-pity, anger and resentment. It's futile to say, "Please stop the world. I want off." You're on "for the duration."

"Why me?" or "why my family?" is the almost universal plaintive query. Jean Marks bravely asserts that the caregiver **must not** become a victim of the disease, and must restructure their own lives. (Aronson et al, pp. 191-192.) I know what the author is saying, but it is still easier to **say** than to **do**.

Having a certain theology or philosophy of life does not necessarily guarantee that your emotions will dutifully follow close behind that theology or philosophy. The knowledge of what you ought to **do** and **be** does not automatically bring with it the power to be and do it. Each of us must find the way.

In the spring of 1987, I was getting near the "ragged edge" and I knew it was time to admit it. The exasperation of having to physically force my Sweetheart to bed and sleep, late at night or in the wee morning hours, pushed me toward the physical and emotional limit. She did not seem to remember or resent it, but it took its toll on me anyway. My "fuse" seemed to get shorter and shorter.

Driving on a precarious road or in heavy traffic with someone distracting you with urgent "directives" can tend to "un-string your banjo." All kinds and grades of stress may contribute toward such a buildup of pain deep inside you. It often takes a long time for real healing to take place.

The first step toward healing is to recognize and admit your limitations and weakness. That is hard for any of us. It collides with our pride head-on. But admit it we must **if** we are ever to find inner wholeness. The next step is to work toward relief from the load you're under.

I thought it was **mostly** *physical* weariness from being "on duty" 24 hours a day for two years. I was wrong. June 1, 1987, came and with it the placing of my Sweetheart in the care of a rest home only eight miles from our home.

"Give me two weeks rest, with a little fishing down at the lake and I'll be my old self again." So I figured.

But it didn't happen. I felt ashamed to admit that I was still bruised, hurt and crushed. I didn't realize how inwardly devastated I was. I needed help and healing. Seeing my Sweetheart desperately straining to keep her identity and personality intact against such overwhelming odds only added to my wounding. We were both cripples. Both sick. We needed help.

Why couldn't we find healing? Had not God come to our rescue with a "healing miracle" when our four children were very young in North Dakota, and delivered Maxine from cancer? And had God not repeated that healing in her when our family was all grown 25 years later at Anderson, Indiana when Brother Loran prayed for her? Both times were real **surprises**, even though we wished, hoped and prayed for it to happen. ("Honest confession...")

Slowly, I began to realize that to be "whole," another healing was sorely needed for both of us. Would it come? If so, what kind of healing, and when?

I Did All I Knew to Do . . .

Faithfully, I gave myself to personal devotions, Scripture reading, and prayer (along with regular church attendance). Twice a day, I went to the nursing home to see Maxine and take her for long walks. With responsibilities at home sharply reduced, I really thought I would be my "old self" again in a couple weeks. But I was not. It seemed that part of what I once was, inside, had died. I tried all I knew to do, and yet I found no healing for my deeper need.

Remembering the sage advice: "When you don't know what to do, just hold steady," I endeavored to do just that – even though I was lonely, and most of life's satisfactions seemed to be gone. Housework, yardwork, worship and visiting my "Maxie" was my routine, while I was still hurting deep inside.

In July, a friend said to me: "Bob, why don't you come go with me to the old camp meeting in Wilmore, Kentucky?"

"Not a bad idea, Ron. I haven't been there for years. I suppose Maxine would make it all right over at the nursing home without me for a few days. Let's do it."

The plans were laid. When time for the camp came, however, Ron was unable to go. But my urge to attend was still with me, so I went alone.

Arriving at Wilmore Camp Meeting late Sunday afternoon, I rented a cot in the men's dorm for a couple nights and attended the evening service in the large tabernacle. The singing was great and the preaching was good, but the crowd of people was disappointingly small. It gave me a lonesome feeling that was depressing. That "special" musty odor of a lumpy cotton mattress that had been brought out of storage for the annual event did not lift my spirits either. The only person there whom I knew was Ralph Blodgett, who was the official "recording" man for the camp.

After a night of very little sleep, I was ready to head back toward Angola, Indiana. I was thinking (or praying): "Lord, if it's OK with You, I'll just check out, head north, and stop in Lexington for breakfast." (I suspect my prayer was more like *telling* God what I planned to do than asking for His suggestions.)

Before I could make my "escape," my friend Ralph came by with a friendly greeting and reminded me of the early morning prayer meeting. Not wanting to seem irreligious, I went with him, thinking: "An hour delay won't hurt anything." But after prayers, Ralph invited me to his room for breakfast. Cereal, milk and fruit finished, we began to reminisce about the 37 years we had served together in the North Indiana Methodist Conference, sharing our joys, sorrows, successes, failures, hopes and dreams. Suddenly, I said, "Hey, Brother, I gotta' go! I'm heading back home to Indiana, like I said."

"Oh, you don't want to head out right now! It's almost time for the morning service. You wouldn't want to miss that, would you, Bob?"

As John Wesley reluctantly went to Aldersgate Street Mission centuries ago in London, so I went to the morning service at the Wilmore Camp Meeting that Monday morning, with renewed determination to head north immediately afterward.

The singing was good and the soloist not bad. The program said the morning speaker was Bishop Henry Ginter, retired, Church of the Brethren, from Pennsylvania. In my experience, many retired Bishops were sort of "over the hill." I was still feeling very low. Lonely. Plain old **depressed**, which was unusual for me. I hadn't seen my Sweetheart for three days now, and I was afraid she would be missing me and forget where I had gone.

I settled back to sleepily listen to the Bishop. He began to speak on a passage from St. Paul's letter to the Church at Philippi. In less than five minutes, I was leaning forward to catch every word. "Hey," I thought, "this old Bishop is still on the 'cutting edge' of things. Sorry, Lord, for misjudging." (Pre-judging, really.)

With rapt attention, I soaked up every word of the sermon, and when he was finished, I was surprised that 40 to 45 minutes had elapsed!

That was six years ago, and as I write these words, my heart floods with gratitude as I remember the inner healing that flowed down to the depths of me on that July morning.

After the service, I said to my friend Ralph, "I want to buy a tape of that sermon so I can listen to it again on the way home."

"I'm already ahead of you, Bob. I'm making a copy as a little gift for you. And say, did you notice that everything the Bishop said this morning seemed to be for you?"

Did I notice! How could I help it? It went from my ears right down inside me. And **God's miracle of deep inner healing began!**

Without the faintest notion of the far-reaching effects of the healing miracle that had begun on that warm Monday morning in July, I said "so long" to Ralph and headed north.

I started for home, "right on schedule." The six hours and many miles to northern Indiana gave time for the sorely needed healing to "settle in" while I listened to Bishop Ginter's message at least twice more from the tape my friend Ralph gave me. I had the cleanest and happiest feeling deep inside that I had enjoyed for several years.

Perhaps you may be saying: "That was more than six years ago. How is it today: Has the process of inner healing continued?"

That's the *best* part! Many great "experiences" seem to be so transitory. The "glow" fades so quickly. But the healing and inner renewal that came to me in July of 1987 has not only continued, but it is getting *better* and *more wonderful* with each passing month and year!

And yet another **"SURPRISE"**! These years have brought a steady renewal and growth of my love for my Sweetheart-wife, Maxine, that is beyond my comprehension. We are now in the seventh year of our "second honeymoon." While her steadily deteriorating physical condition pains me greatly, the JOY of belonging to her and **our** belonging to God floods in so steadily that it drives the pain right out of me.

A big part of that JOY is the close-up view of her yet *unchanged Christian personality.* Though I have heard her speak only one word since January 1, 1990, she says volumes with those beautiful eyes and her cooperative attitude and spirit. One of the last sentences I remember hearing her say was to a little elderly lady on a walker as we were breezing down the hall. As we passed, she reached over and patted her hand. Looking back over her shoulder, she cheerily called, "I love you!" That was – and is – my "Maxie"!

"Wings to soar the heights" it seems we have been given while we joyfully walk together on earth. Just **incredible**! Yet, every word of what I'm trying to tell you is true!

Dr. Martin Luther King, Jr., would say, "I've been to the mountain top, children! And there's **GLORY** up there!"

*   *   *

There are many mysteries about this "mountain." But a few things I think I understand already: The way **up** is made possible only by "mercy" and "grace" from God. But must we not do something? Yes, if you want to call **receptivity** and **response** doing something. But trusting and obeying seem to be such a tiny "minimum response" for such great benefits of **"glory"** we experience on the way up the mountain!

*   *   *

Many of the nurses and aides at Grace Village seem to catch glimpses of the **glory** Maxine and I enjoy as we walk the halls. "Here come those lovers," they often say. Since Maxine doesn't talk, I have to do it all. But she can ask someone's name just by a certain look she gives me.

We have about one-half mile of halls at Grace Village. One round trip is a mile. We were doing about two miles a day, but now she walks slower and not nearly as far. Call me a "mystic" if you wish, but many times there is the exhilerating sense that we are not walking alone.

*   *   *

So we walk and I talk and sing. Since my selection is limited and I don't want to bore her with repeats, I just make up songs as we go. Sometimes singing in cadence with our steps. Truly original songs, never sung before by mortal man nor heard by mortal woman!

We have fun. More than that, we have JOY.

Better yet, we have a **GLORY!** I suppose Max Lucado would call this joy, fun and glory "holy jewels quarried out of the mine of despair." The descriptive phrase is so accurate! (See Lucado.)

Like the deep inner healing at the old campground at Wilmore, Kentucky. **God often does most wonderful things in the most unlikely places!** His timing often surprises us too. You can't "program" a soverign God. Yet you can always *depend* on this: God consistently **comes to us**, meeting us at the point of our greatest need, again and again.

". . . to Bind Up the Brokenhearted . . ."

To me, Isaiah 61:1-3 is one of the most accurate and beautiful prophecies to be found anywhere in the Old Testament: "The Spirit of the Sovereign Lord is on me, because He has sent me to **bind up the brokenhearted**, to proclaim freedom for the captives, and release for the prisoners, to proclaim the year of the Lord's favor and the day of vengeance of our God, to comfort all who mourn, and provide for those who grieve in Zion – to bestow on them a crown of beauty instead of ashes, the oil of gladness instead of mourning, and **a garment of praise instead of** *a spirit of despair.* They will be called oaks of righteousness, a planting of the Lord for the display of his splendor." (Bold & italics are mine for emphasis.)

* * *

Looking back six or eight years and comparing "the garment of praise" we enjoy now with the tight grip the "spirit of despair" had on Maxine and me, I keep asking: "How could this deliverance, help, and healing – this **glory** have happened to us? To me?

This question also keeps coming: "How can I say 'Thanks' adequately, for all He's done for me?" I plan to keep right on looking for the answer to that last question.

André Crouch has put that question so beautifully in the lyrics to his beloved song. Why not review it?

HOW CAN I SAY THANKS?

How can I say thanks for the things
    You have done for me?
Things so undeserved,
    Yet you gave to prove Your love for me;
The voices of a million angels
    Could not express my gratitude,
All that I am, and ever hope to be,
    I owe it all to Thee.

To God be the glory! To God be the glory!
    To God be the glory, for the things
He has done!
    With His blood He has saved me;
With His power He has raised me;
    To God be the glory for the things He has done!

Just let me live my life,
    Let it be pleasing, Lord, to Thee;
And if I gain any praise,
    Let it go to Calvary.

With His blood He has saved me;
    With His power He has raised me;
To God be the glory
    For the things He has done!

Our thanks to you, André, for your willingness to be an "open channel" of inspiration to help us all express the gratitude bubbling out of our hearts.

*   *   *

We hear about "Going for the Gold," We are proud of those just returning from Lillehammer, Norway, who excelled. Those who "bring home the gold" comprise quite an exclusive club. But there is a price to be paid **for** and **by** each one who become winners. That price is beyond the reach of most of us. Participation via "spectatorship" is as close as most of us will ever get to the **gold**. And that's OK in many things.

But what if *the world's best kept secret* should begin to leak out that **each of us** can have a **"glory"**? What if it really **is** a true word: The Creator of us all shows no partiality? Then those who have a **"glory"** deep inside (many in spite of a bunch of agonizing reverses) are not special at all, but have just opened themselves up to what was coming down for everyone all along?

Have you ever been to a "mountain top"? How did you get there? What did you see on top? Was it worth the effort? Silly question! Anyone who has ever been held a willing captive of a **glory** knows the answer is "YES"! A thousand times over!

To you brave souls who long to breathe the exhilarating air of the "mountain top," let me review just a few of the "watchwords" you perhaps already know as sign posts along the way up.

Humility. You can't go **up** until first you go **down** in true humbleness of heart. If you think you can handle everything yourself, you're doomed to try it.

Trust. Not in luck, circumstances, or fate, but in the one true and living God.

Faithfulness. Persistence is within the reach of each of us. Faithfulness takes no special talents, or special endowments. We can each keep on keeping on.

Integrity. If you really want to *"Go for the Glory,"* then learn the meaning of this great word, and apply it to all your relationships in life. You can't find a substitute for it.

Each of us have a perfect right to our own personal faith. I respect yours, and hope you grant me the same courtesy. I have become vulnerable in exposing to you just a wee glimpse of my experience. I'm still growing, and hope you are too. My faith includes fun and humor. I invite you into the next chapter for a brief exploration of it.

THROUGH IT ALL

Keeping – and Using – A Sense of Humor

IT MAY BE POSSIBLE to get along without a sense of humor, but you can get along a lot better with it! That goes for good times and bad. But it's even more important in difficult times. Proverbs 17:22 says:

"A cheerful heart is good medicine,
but a crushed spirit dries up the bones." *(NIV)*

That must have been what Nehemiah had in mind as he comforted the repentant, mourning people at Jerusalem a long time ago. He said to them:

"Do not grieve, for the **joy of the Lord**
is your strength." *(Nehemiah 8:10 b, NIIV)*
(Bold is author's for imphasis)

If you say, "I'm trusting God," then you should be an optimist with a sense of humor. A vital faith prevents pessimism. The two are mutually exclusive. You cannot be a trusting soul with reservations and doubt.

"Trusting" people are cheerful; optimistic. Hopeful people can see humor in situations where others choose to allow troubles and difficulties to blind them.

Times of mourning, sorrow and weeping come to all of us. But the "motif" of the symphony of our life can be one of **joy** and good humor. Optimism. We need to laugh a whole sight more than we cry. That, I believe, is one of the secrets of going through difficult, harrowing experiences and "coming out in one piece" or a "whole" person.

A long time ago I heard it said: "God can pull you through anything if you'll just stick together while He's pulling." I believe a wholesome sense of humor is part of the "glue" that helps us stick together while God pulls!

> "A happy heart makes the face cheerful,
> but heartache crushes the spirit.
> The discerning heart seeks knowledge,
> but the mouth of a fool **feeds on folly**."
> *(Proverbs 15:13-14 NIV)*

All of chapter 15 is so excellent in the bold contrasts depicted, let me quote two more verses from it:

> "A gentle answer turns away wrath,
> but a harsh word stirs up anger.
> The tongue of the wise commends knowledge,
> but the mouth of the fool **gushes folly**."
> *(Proverbs 15:1-2, NIV* – emphasis mine)

This does not negate good, wholesome fun and laughter. A careful look at Ecclesiastes 7:6 will help.

> "Like the crackling of thorns under the pot,
> so is the laughter of fools.
> This, too, is meaningless."

Meaningless is a key word. Sometimes you can lighten up a very "heavy" situation with a bit of humor.

Like the day one lady (let's call her Sue) who was giving the nurses and aides "fits." Nobody could do or say anything to please her. The food looked great to me, but refusing even to taste it, she began calling it uncomplimentary names (along with anyone who dared suggest she take at least a little bite of it). In an effort to relieve the tension, I jokingly said: "Sue, why are you being **so difficult**? With just a **little more effort**, you could be absolutely impossible!"

Everyone within earshot had a good laugh – except Sue. Still sulking, she finally remarked: "I didn't see anything funny about that." Well, I tried. At least it relieved the tension.

My friend Harold Williams, with his sense of humor and fun stories, adds so much to all our lives at the Village. I asked him one day if he thought even God had a sense of humor. "You want proof?" said he. "Just look at a bunch of people, or take a careful look in the mirror and remember **God made us all!**"

To Laugh or to Cry . . .

There are times and situations when you don't know whether to laugh or to cry. I choose laughter because it seems positive and optimistic. "Laugh and the world laughs with you; cry and you cry alone" has a lot of truth in it. Laughter is, I believe, one of God's good gifts to us. Yet, we must choose to accept and use the gift.

Some years ago at a busy restaurant several of us were in line at the cashier. My wife Maxine broke from the line, circled back to the table we had left, and deftly retrieved the $3.00 tip – just ahead of the astounded waitress.

Quietly moving toward them, I gently took the money from her and gave it to the puzzled waitress. "She has Alzheimer's, I quietly explained. The look on the waitress' face turned from distress to understanding, relief, and *finally to a grateful smile.* The quick changes on her face were so comical!

With a light little chuckle, she said, "Thank you so, much. Come back now!"

We Even Have Fun Over in the Health Care Unit!

Spending many hours in Health Care feeding my "Maxie" and taking her for walks the past seven years has furthered my education in that field considerably. Understanding more fully tends to make one more tolerant and less judgmental. I hope this sharing will be interesting, enlightening and help in the development of your sense of humor.

*   *   *

▲ I noticed that this one lady almost **always** had her "trouble light" on. It was easy to see that the nurses and aides did not usually "rush" to answer it. One day I said to the nurse: "I notice that Suzie **almost always** has her light on."

"Yes, came the weary reply. "All day long she

wants to go to the bathroom every ten minutes. And the results are always predictable. Nil." Then I understood the occasional "slowness" of response on the part of the aides.

One day I passed by Suzie's door and had a shock. Her trouble light was **not** on! Seeing several nurses and aides near the nurses' station, I said excitedly: "Come, girls! Let us 'kill the fatted chicken' and celebrate!" When I had their attention, I asked: "Do you see what I see? Look!" When they began to wonder about **me**, I added: "Haven't you noticed? **Suzie's light is not on!**"

"Ohoooo!" they all exclaimed. "There's a first time for everything!" We all had a good laugh. Experience teaches, albeit quite slowly at times, the old "Wolf! Wolf!" story we learned as children is still with us, and needed.

It is possible for one's spirit to get hardened in a health care place, but I'm thankful to report that **most** of the people I've known these seven years are very **caring** people.

▲ How I wish each of you had a mental picture I carry with me of this BIG man who resembled a lineman from the Chicago Bears squad. As a **volunteer** he was helping feed those not able to feed themselves. He was doing it with such patience and tenderness that I neglected my Maxine for several seconds just to watch him! I wanted to meet and talk with him after the meal, but it didn't work out. The **contrast** of his size and muscular build to the little old lady he was feeding would have been hilariously funny, if I had not been so captivated with his *gentleness.* I thought to myself "Now there is a real gentle man." I wish he would come back soon!

*   *   *

A bit of poetry a college professor shared with us years ago pretty well sums up my feeling about life.

> This world is filled so full of joys
> Which little woes can ne'er destroy,
> What if one trouble comes my way?
> I'll smile at it and simply say,
> "Of one fair blessing I'm bereft,
> But, oh! I have a million left."

Life has its times of weeping and sorrow. We may focus on them if we choose, and eventually our "record" will get stuck in that monotonous groove. But we may choose an attitude of faith/optimism. It says: "We can make it through whatever comes. Even death."

We weep, but not without hope. Hope and faith tell us "**joy** comes in the morning." That attitude is a stabilizing and driving force if we embrace it. A basic sense of humor may help to lift, energize, and get you through serious situations even when no laughter seems possible or appropriate.

*   *   *

▲ Yesterday in Health Care, I noticed that Maxine's glasses had a name taped on the temple piece. (And they were not hers. Maxine's has her initials in gold on the lense) The nurse went with me to the neighbor across the hall. Sure enough, she was wearing Maxine's! We diplomatically traded with her. This same neighbor started into Maxine's room later that day and I said, "No dear, your room is across the hall there! See, there is your name and picture by the door!"

"Yes, I know" she reluctantly admitted. "That's my

bedroom, but this other room across the hall is mine, too. That's where I entertain my guests." Then I knew how the eyeglasses got switched! The nurses and aides had a laugh. But little surprises them.

▲ Some time ago in the Health Care dining room, Bertha and another lady were standing around waiting for dinner. They were engaged in animated conversation, toe to toe, It was apparent to us who were listening that they were not on the same topic. Furthermore, neither had any continuity in what they were individually saying. Finally, Bertha paused, put her hands on her hips and said, "Oh, dear! I'm all mixed up!"

I began to chuckle, and said: "Don't worry about it, Bertha. You're still far ahead. At least you realize it. Just think of all the people in the world who are all mixed up and don't even know it!"

▲ A few years ago Maxine wanted a new pair of dress shoes. I went up town and bought her a nice pair of red ones "on trial." I took them to the nursing home, tried them on, and they fit perfectly! And she loved them! So delighted. She said to me: "I'm saving **these** for Sunday. I have plenty of older ones for everyday."

I told her I thought it was a good idea. The next day when I went a little earlier to take her for a walk, she was still in bed. "Hey, kid, why are you still in bed? Let's take a walk, OK?

Pulling back the covers revealed that she still had on pajamas, but also her new red shoes! Just then a nurse came in. I must have had a quizzical look on my face.

Quickly, she said with a giggle, "You know, last night she wouldn't let us take off those new shoes! Since they were new and clean, we thought it would do no harm to humor her and let her sleep in them"

We all thought that was a cute one, Funny, really. But it has so much **sweetness** in it that I still laugh, and end up with a few tears. How I love that girl! If I had to choose a life mate again, knowing all I know now, I would still choose her without a moment's hesitation.

Guardian Angels?

Happily visiting with nurses and aides before starting down the hall for our pre-lunch walk, Maxine and I turned to go. In a fraction of a second I discovered that my hold on her arm was not as secure as I thought. Down she went to the floor, with nurses and aides all joining me in a desperate, though futile, grab for her. She seemed to be OK., so we raised her to her feet and away we went for our walk.

But before leaving, I looked at my gracious helpers and said: "Don't anyone ever say you don't believe in **guardian angels**! That makes about 69 times (a slight exaggeration) she has fallen in the last six months, **with no injury or bruises**, even!" With an ever-deepening gratitude, we proceeded down the hall on one of our "little dates" as Maxine used to call them.

To avoid an attitude of being **presumptuous** (as we are taught in Matthew 4:6-7) , I am now careful to use the web safety belt provided for us, while still being so very grateful for the constant ministry of the Lord's "guardian angels" promised in Psalm 91:11-12.

I suspect that for millions of us in "the discipline of the difficult," one Bible verse that stands high in the "favorites" list is I Corinthians 10:13. I especially like this one in the Amplified Version, by Zondervan:

"For no temptation – no trial regarded as enticing to sin (no matter how it comes or where it leads) – has overtaken you and laid hold on you that is not common to man – that is, no temptation or trial has come to you that is beyond human resistance and that is not adjusted and adapted and belonging to human experience, and such as man can bear. But God is faithful (to His Word and to His compassionate nature), and He (can be trusted) not to let you be tempted and tried and assayed beyond your ability and strength to endure, but with the temptation He will (always) also **provide the way out** – the means of escape to a landing place – that you may be capable and strong and powerful patiently to bear up under it."

Isn't that great? It would **not** be if it were not **true.** But **millions** of us, with one voice, say:

"Yes! It is both **beautiful** and **true!**"

* * *

No matter how old you are or what your condition is, I hope you are optimistic and have a sense of humor. It is good for your liver, digestive system, heart – and all the rest of your body – to say nothing of the "real **you**" that inhabits the body! Besides helping you, it will help everyone around you or related in any way to you.

* * *

As nature rejects a vacuum, so it seems to me, our human nature cannot tolerate the thought of having lived without **making a difference** (at least a small one) in the world while we're here. Choosing, by faith, an attitude of hope and cheerfulness will make it **certain** that we will be making a **good difference** while we live and a legacy of great value to leave after we're gone. So may it be!

8

CAREGIVER DISTRESS

Helping the Family

by CAROL J. VAN PELT, MSN

THIS CENTURY has witnessed an EXPLOSION of **knowledge** that surpasses all the preceding 19 combined. The breakthrough in the sharing of information, and especially that of technology, can be a "boon or a bust" to our nation and to the whole human race – depending on how we channel and use that knowledge.

Conservation is a word that must become BIG with meaning to us and our world. The multiplicity of **needs** among us humans at this very moment is staggering; needs enough to tax the brain power and soul power of every one of us in the great adventure of **meeting** those needs.

Hence, we need to be concerned about **waste**. I do not mean the mounting tons of garbage that no one can figure out where to safely deposit but the tragic waste of human life.

Every youth who gets hooked on drugs is a part of that colossal waste. Every person who is "under-employed" or unemployed is part of that waste. Every senator and every local citizen who gets ethically and morally "derailed" is a part of that tragic drain on our priceless national moral capital. Every life and every dollar lost to crime is a terrible prodigality that no nation can afford to tolerate.

The need of the hour is people of all ages who will commit themselves to be a part of the **answer** rather than a part of the world's problems.

Health Care Reform is on the American mind. We have the knowledge. We have the potential to supply the health needs of every person in the nation. Our problem now is how to get the medicine to "where it hurts" and apply it.

Perhaps you noticed on your TV screen the "FACTOID" some time ago: *"54% of Americans surveyed said they would be willing to receive their primary medical care from a nurse with a Masters degree rather than a M.D."*

That may be indicative of the direction we need to go if the dream of adequate medical care for every citizen is to become reality in this generation.

Since I graduating from Indiana University with a Master of Science in Nursing (MSN) degree, let me share with you in this chapter a bit of the wealth of information uncovered in writing just **one** paper for **one** class. You determined souls who wade through the chapter, and then review what you have read, may find an index to a wealth of helpful information on **one** part of **one** of our BIG problems: Caregiver stress in families with ADRD (Alzheimer's disease and related dementia).

For those of you who may not realize the magnitude of the problem, let me share an extensive quote from a newspaper *(Times-Union,* Warsaw, Indiana) dated January 18, 1994:

CHICAGO (AP) – Nearly half of all Americans have a psychiatric disorder at some time in their lives, usually depression, problem drinking or some kind of phobia, researchers say. Nearly 30 percent are afflicted in any given year, say researchers who conducted the most extensive U.S. survey of its kind in a decade.

"The researchers said mental disorders were found to be more common than previously believed, and more needs to be learned about why many people don't seek help.

"It shouldn't be scary to say half the population has suffered some mental disorder. That's part of life," said lead researcher Ronald C. Kessler, a sociology professor at the University of Michigan.

"Researchers looked for 14 of the most common mental illnesses. Forty-eight percent of the 8,098 respondents had at least one disorder at some time during their lives; 29.5 percent had been afflicted within the previous 12 months.

"An important discovery was that 79 percent of cases of mental illness are concentrated in a small proportion of people – 14 percent of the population – with multiple psychiatric problems. . . . The trick is to figure out the nature of the pileups . . . before people crawl into the psychiatrist's office divorced and alcoholic," he said.

That quote may give you a clue as to the extent of mental illness with which we must deal. In this chapter our scope is narrowed to ADRD and related caregiver stress.

I agree with what my father has said earlier in this book. The time has come for civilized people to cease making jokes about mental illness/diseases of the brain and begin to take seriously the prevention of brain diseases, along with treatment and care of those already afflicted. Really now, why should a brain disease bring a social stigma any more than heart disease? Who makes jokes about people with heart trouble or cancer?

Alzheimer's disease and related dementias (ADRD) account for one of the largest groups causing caregiver distress. A report by Brady & Cohen (1989), revealed that there were approximately 27 million people 65 years and older at that time. They projected that by the year 2000 there will be 50-60 million people 65 and older. Brady & Cohen also reported that according to Roth (cited in Hay & Ernst 1987), by the year 2050 there will be more than 8.5 million people with ADRD. A positive way to look at it would be to say that of these 50-60 million older people, 83 percent to 86 percent of them will **not** have any dementia! And we all hope and pray to be in **that** number!

An ADRD patient can live anywhere from one to 20 years after diagnosis, depending on other concurrent illnesses. It is staggering to multiply those numbers by the billions of dollars that must be set aside for the care of persons with ADRD alone. The government, no doubt, will look at the numbers and try to find a way to reduce them. One of the more obvious ways is to postpone institutionalization by promoting care in the home by the family. In that case, we will need more funding for additional help for families, which translates into additional funding and practitioners trained and willing to assist.

This review will look first at the family in regard to caregiving. Next, the idea of caregiver distress will be studied as it applies to families and caring for ADRD patients. And finally, implications for advanced nursing practice.

Family As Caregiver

Webster defines family as (1) all the people living in the same house; (2) parents and children; (3) relatives, and (4) all those descended from a common ancestor. Others see the family as people that meet each other's needs.

Reutter (1984) sees the family system as having two main tasks. The first is to meet the "self-care requirements of air, food, water, elimination, rest and activity; and the second is adapting to change" (p 394). An additional family task of supporting each member through the changing life stages and providing loving, non-judgmental care in whatever way is needed, is seen as vital by this writer.

One amazing family attribute is the diverse ways families find to provide care for their needy members. At one time there was an impression that families were abandoning their elders to institutions in alarming numbers. It appeared that families did not want to care for elders who were something of a bother. However, when the research was done, the **opposite** was found! Peters, Hoyt, Babchuk, Kaiser & Iijma (1987) reported a large number of contacts between elders and their extended families. At least half the elderly reported seeing at least one child per day and a third reported seeing a sibling each week. Family members provide at least 80 percent of care given to aging members (Ory, 1985).

Caregivers are primarily spouses, if there is one. If the spouse is unavailable, then adult children take over the primary role (Ory 1985. Normally one person assumes the primary caregiver role (Deimling et al 1989; Ory, 1985; and Peters et al). Although 85 percent of caregivers are women (Braithwaite, 1992; Ory, 1985), the contribution that men make in caring for their wives should not be overlooked. There are fewer men caregivers in number, but that is probably due in part to the relatively shorter life span of men. Male and female caregivers both face the isolation and exhaustion of providing care at home.

Because caregiving was seen as a private family matter, caregiver distress was long overlooked and ignored. Women were expected to accept the caregiver role as part of their family duties and were expected to continue doing it as long as necessary. Sommers (1985) explained the "compassion trap": Women as a group have always been helpers. They respond to needs in other people and are thus willing to take on tasks that are exhausting and often undervalued by other family members. To many, the word "family" really means "closest female relative" (p 10).

Caregiver Distress

Caregiver distress has been defined in a number of ways. George & Gwyther (1986) described it as "the physical, psychological or emotional, social, and financial problems that can be experienced by family members caring for impaired older adults" (p 253). Ory (1985) says "burden (distress) may be defined as the impact of the changes in cognition and behavior of the patient and family, and the patient's subsequent need for care and supervision" (p 631).

As interest in distress was sparked, further research was undertaken to aid understanding of **how** the caregiver became distressed, the degree of distress in various settings (Braithwaite 1992; Deimling et al 1989; and Moritz et al 1992), the **effects** of distress on the caregiver (Romeis 1989; and Tennstedt, Cafferata & Sullivan (1992) and how distress relates to public policy (Braithwaite 1992).

Effects of Distress on Caregiver and Family

Caregiver distress has been shown to affect the family in many ways. First, the caregiver may suffer physically. Stress in the form of depression is the most common form of distress (Tennstedt et al, 1992). The stress is almost universal in occurrence, but the disabling aspects of stress vary a great deal. Since each family may feel the stress differently, depending on whether they view caring for the person as a chore or a privilege, the stress can be seen as either positive or negative. Moritz et al (1992) reported that men caring for impaired spouses were more susceptible to significant increases in blood pressure. Especially if the distress is perceived in a negative way, the caregiver may find herself/himself unable to continue in the role of primary caregiver.

The next area of possible conflict is in the area of **employment**. If the caregiver is female, other family members may not view her employment as important and pressure her to quit her job. If she values the job but is having problems at work, she may give in to the family wishes but be resentful. If the caregiver is a male, his employment will probably be seen as essential and the family will eventually find another solution.

An area closely related to employment is that of **financial burden**. If the caregiver has given up a job to care for the family member, the lost income can place additional stress on the caregiver family as well as place added stress on the caregiver/care-receiver relationship. Families find that *in no way does Medicare/Medicaid absorb all the costs involved,* and thus the person paying the bills can incur significant out-of-pocket expenses.

Personal disruptions can account for a significant part of distress encountered by the caregiver. Adult children who take on the caregiving responsibilities of a parent or family member with ADRD also have responsibilities in their own home. They often have a spouse and children who also require care and attention. They are the ones that can get left behind. The caregiver's family may need time and help of their own and feel that the care-receiver is getting all the available resources. This can cause bitterness and ultimately, rifts in the family. If the spouse of the caregiver is unhappy with the situation, it could put the marriage at risk (Adamson et al 1992).

Another part of personal disruptions is the situation where the care-receiver is brought **into the caregiver's home**. Especially if the patient requires help during the night, wake and sleep times may be disrupted for the entire family. The caregiver may have difficulty getting back to sleep once interrupted, and become exhausted after a short time. It is common for ADRD patients to suffer from sleep disturbances. If awake during the night, the caregiver must be awake too, to ensure that the patient does not go outside the house and wander off. The care-receiver may be able to "cat nap" during the day, but the caregiver must be alert all the time.

Social isolation can be one of the most devastating parts of being a caregiver. Friends come to visit for a time, but visits may be uncomfortable and, therefore, cease after a while. The caregiver may be hesitant to ask for help from other family members. Or the family may not want to intrude on the caregiver's "turf." The patient may not want the caregiver to leave him/her with anyone else or be left alone and may become frantic when even discussing it. Guilt feelings often forces the caregiver to give up ideas of self enjoyment. As the caregiver decreases contact with the community, friends stop attempting to get the caregiver involved in activities. Before long the opportunities are gone (Brubaker 1987; Culter 1985). At times it is easier to stay home than to create upset.

Privacy and time alone for the caregiver and spouse can be another area for discord. Any unresolved conflicts can re-surface and spoil the harmony. If all the energy that was once spent maintaining the marriage relationship is now spent on caregiving tasks, the marriage will suffer.

Physical abuse is another topic that is frequently mentioned by dementia caregivers. The patient may have extreme changes in personality that include verbal and physical abuse. It is equally possible that the frustrations inherent in caring for an ADRD patient could bring the caregiver to verbally or physically abuse the patient.

Taking on the caregiver role may mean that the
child is now caring for the parent. **Role reversal** can
be very distressing. If the previous relationship was
close, the caregiver may feel she/he is intruding into
private areas. If the relationship was not close, the
caregiver may feel the need to make up for that by
agreeing to be the primary caregiver.

The last area for discussion is the distress caused
by **having to make decisions**. The primary
caregiver may feel that since she/he is doing all the
work, then she/he should make all the decisions. Or,
the primary caregiver may not **want** to make any
decisions. Knowing that a steady stream of decisions must be made by someone only increases the
caregiver distress.

Implications for Nursing Practice

Because Alzheimer's disease and related dementia
(ADRD) is a common problem, the Nurse Practitioner
(NP) will inevitably be involved with clients with
ADRD. It will be important to begin interventions as
early as possible in order to assist the family unit
promptly.

Once the diagnosis has been made, if the client or
family is wishing to return to your care, the NP must
decide if she/he is ready, willing and able to accept the
client and family in a very time and energy intensive
case management role (Eisdorfer, Rabins & Reisberg
1991).

If the NP accepts the role of case manager, it is
best to start with a meeting of as many of the client's
family members as possible. Either one long or several shorter meetings will need to be scheduled. Review with them their understanding of the diagnosis,
disease progression, and prognosis. Any misunder-

standings should be corrected and the family directed to additional reading if needed (Eisdorfer et al 1991).

Meeting with as many members of the family as possible gives the NP an opportunity to discuss the stresses involved in caring for an ADRD patient. It is an ideal time to encourage working together and sharing of the tremendous burden. Because the burden will become heavier in the future, it gives the family a chance to work together and get some practice before that time.

The meeting also gives the NP an opportunity to observe the family dynamics. It is important to know how each family member feels about the situation, and how much they are committed to helping. The cultural norms must also be understood by the practitioner. This is an excellent time to encourage the family to seek a financial and a legal advisor in order to clarify ownership and guardianship issues (Eisdorfer et al 1991).

Client families may become discouraged with confusing or conflicting information from government agencies. It is important to encourage families in their quest for assistance or simply for answers. At times, only persistence finally leads them to the people who can answer their questions and ultimately help them. The NP must resist the urge to solve all problems for the family. It is more important to show them the right direction and support them in their quest.

The nurse must be on the alert for symptoms of depression (especially insomnia, loss of appetite, and weight loss) and substance abuse. Primary caregivers are especially at risk, due to the stress involved (Eisdorfer et al 1991).

During routine visits it is important that the practitioner question the primary caregiver(s) about **respite breaks**. Are the other family members giving the primary caregiver time away from the client on a regular basis. Sometimes the caregiver refuses the offers, or is unwilling to ask for help. the family must understand that in order to be effective, the caregiver must have time for personal activities (Eisdorfer et al 1991; Pallett 1990).

Encourage the family to find a support group. If possible, keep a notebook of current community groups active in your area so that a phone number can be readily available.

Dealing with caregiver negative emotions can be one of the hardest subjects to deal with for the NP. **Guilt** is the number one emotion in caregivers of ADRD patients. Guilt is very destructive because the caregiver may *make choices based on a feeling of guilt and not on what is best for the person and the family* at that particular time (Eisdorfer et al 1991).

The second most common negative emotion is **anger**. It is helpful to reinforce with the caregiver that it is the disease that causes the patient to act the way he/she does, and that the patient has no control over it. If the caregiver will talk about the feelings, it is the beginning of dealing with them. Be aware that anger that gets out of bounds can lead to abuse. Any situation of abuse must be treated immediately with **respite care** for the caregiver (Eisdorfer et al 1991). My dad recalls that he noticed that his "fuse" was getting "shorter and shorter" in spite of the fact that he had regular respite care four hours each week. He sought relief by placing our mother in a nursing home. My sister and I fully supported him and encouraged him in that need.

Since most ADRD patients require nursing home care eventually, it is good to bring up the subject early in the course of the disease. If certain family members are opposed to the idea,it gives the practitioner time to explore the reasons for the resistance (Eisdorfer et al 1991).

After the death of your ADRD patient, the NP might consider one last meeting with the family members to allow for ventilation of feelings. It also allows the practitioner to obtain closure in the relationship with the family that may have extended for many years (Eisdorfer et al 1991).

In addition to dealing with the client and family, the NP must consider public policy. Nursing research needs to look at the best way to help families deal with an ADRD patient at home, to obtain respite and institutional care without becoming destitute in the process, and then pass along the information to the government agencies.

Conclusions

The care of ADRD patients and the distress that is encountered by families has far-reaching effects on our society. As the population ages and people live longer, more cases of ADRD will be experienced by families. Nurse Practitioners will also be managing their care. Nurses must be knowledgeable not only about the disease but about how to help families through it. In this chapter, we have looked at families, distress, how distress affects family functioning, and implications for nursing practice. Nursing must not sit on their collective hands and bewail their fate. There is research that needs to be done in order to convince government agencies that nurses have ideas about caring for clients and can carry them out successfully. Nurses can handle prescriptive authority and use it wisely. Nurses have the skill and ability to care for ADRD clients and make a difference in this monumental task.

We need to accept the challenge presented by the explosion of knowledge and the opportunities presented by this age of **communication**. The people who will make the real difference will be those daring souls committed to the **EXPLOSION OF CARING** right in the middle of an egocentric, self-serving generation that often seems bent only on what they want. Let me challenge you to a deep determination to start right where you are and be part of the **answer** to the fast-multiplying physical, mental and spiritual needs of our society rather than a part of the problem.

Rabbi Harold S. Kushner has said it so well, I want to quote him:

> "God inspires people to help other people who have been hurt by life, and by helping them, they protect them from the danger of feeling alone, abandoned, or judged. God makes some people want to become doctors and nurses, to spend days and nights of self-sacrificing concern with an intensity for which no money can compensate, in the effort to sustain life and alleviate pain. God moves people to want to be medical researchers, to focus their intelligence and energy on the causes and possible cures for some of life's tragedies. . . . God, who neither causes nor prevents tragedies, helps by inspiring people to help" (Rabbi H. S. Kushner, ibid).

I am committed to the belief that life is good, worth living and worth conserving (saving). Being a "committee of one" to **serve** in a "give me" generation can bring a feeling of loneliness at times. But it also has its great satisfactions and deep **joys**! You know you are not "on your on" nor are you ever alone. With confidence I tell you what I know every member of our family will joyfully confirm.

Mom was diagnosed with AD more than nine years ago. As we took a backward look, we could see that it started ten years before that time. Dad retired two years early. We two daughters and our husbands pitched in to help him lovingly care for her. The obvious **joy** that remains in their wonderful marriage is an inspiration to us and to a wide circle of friends and acquaintances. They have proved that the "in spite of" brand of true happiness **does still exist**!

Our word to you who share a bit of their story via this book is that **joy** is for **everyone** – *in spite of everything!*

As individuals and as a family, we have **tested** the promises found in Isaiah 41:10 and Matthew 28:20, along with many others.

Senior Statistics

- Since 1985, there have been more Americans over age 65 than under age 18.

- There are more Americans over age 65 than the entire population of Canada.

- There are approximately 40,000 Americans over 100 years old.

- Over one-fourth of all men over age 55 and one-half of men over age 62 are retired.

- The vast majority of retirees do not move when they retire.

- Over 60% of all single adults are older people.

- By 2040, the average life expectancy for men will be 87 years and 92 years for women.

THE HUMAN TOUCH

Caregiving As Seen From Inside A Health Care Facility

by DARLENE ROHRER,
Assistant Director of Nursing
Grace Village Health Care
Winona Lake, Indiana

WHETHER OR NOT we have had occasion to visit one, we have all heard something about the health care institutions once known as "rest homes." Much of what we heard was uncomplimentary. Some were even horror stories.

Many, if not most, have changed their names. Now they call themselves "Happy Days Health Care Center" or? The names have changed but that's not all, fortunately, for millions of the elderly. Often at the stubborn prodding of governmental agencies, both the smell and the quality of caregiving have improved considerably. The battle for excellence still goes on, however.

Here in Winona Lake, Indiana, we are so fortunate as to have a splendid Christian retirement facility called "Grace Village." Connected with it is Grace

Village Health Care, which we think has also developed into one of the better ones in this part of the state. (Not perfect yet, but making a real push in that direction!) Mr. Boggs has an apartment in Grace Village Retirement Complex of which the Health Care is a part. Thus, he is able to take Maxine for walks in the halls in safety and comfort summer and winter.

Many of the things people know about "rest homes" is quite vague and faceless, with workers often depicted as hard and uncaring. Mr. Boggs thought it might be good for me to give you a glimpse of caregiving as seen – and felt – from inside an institution by at least one of the many who labor at the task of caregiving.

*   *   *

How well I remember the day Rev. and Mrs. Boggs walked through the front doors of the nursing home. Their faces looked familiar, but I just couldn't remember where I had met them.

Arm in arm they walked up to the nurses station and Mr. Boggs introduced his Maxine as our new resident. You could see the love in his eyes for her. But you could also feel hurt and a bit of hesitation in his voice at the prospect of entrusting her care to yet another group of strangers.

I asked him where they were from and he told me they had been serving as pastor and wife in churches of the North Indiana Conference of the United Methodists since 1952. I suddenly remembered that it was at pastors meetings and youth camps I had seen them several years back.

As we walked Maxine to her room, she clung silently to her husband's arm. In her room we began showing them how to operate the bed and the call light. Mr. Boggs interrupted:

"But my 'Maxie' won't remember to use the call light."

How my heart ached for him as I remembered taking my own mentally retarded son to a home for handicapped children. I felt that no one could possibly love him or care for him like I could. but I also knew it was a 24-hour job.

In my heart, I wanted to try to let Mr. Boggs know that we would do our very best to care for his Sweetheart wife and keep her safe. I assured him that we have a "nurse alert" cord that we pin to her clothing so that if she became restless and tried to get up, it would pull the call light on and staff would come to assist her.

As time passed, we have shared what Maxine could still do for herself and the things she liked to do; like playing the piano, reading and walking. Playing the piano and reading both faded out after about a year. Two years later, she quit trying to talk. But for three and one-half years she is still able to eat well and take two walks each day with her husband.

We on the staff have what we call "Care Plan" meetings with the family. Early on, Mr. Boggs explained that Maxine's short attention span made it impossible for her to carry through on any projects, except listening to gospel music and watching television. She loves to eat, he said, but has to have constant prompting and reminders to slow down. I will mention later how valuable a bit of information that was!

Let me mention that first day again. As I was getting Maxine settled into her room, Mr. Boggs began bringing in her personal items to make it seem more familiar to her. You could see the twinkle in her eyes as she watched him go in and out of the room. I knew how he must be torn by emotion upon entering this new phase of their changing lives here at Grace Village.

From the inside some of us get a pretty clear picture of the broad spectrum of people and their family life and backgrounds. As time has passed our staff have come to admire Mr. Boggs' devotion to his wife. With all the broken marriages in our society around us, the Boggs have been a real inspiration to all of us. Even though Maxine does not speak any more, you can see her love returned in a smile or the tender kiss she always has for her husband when he comes to her. If you could have been here with the approximately 300 people to help them celebrate their 50th wedding anniversary on July 10, you would have been deeply touched as he sang to her "I Love You Truly."

I believe it has been this devotion between them that has kept Maxine walking so well these past six years. Our staff walks her daily to meals and activities; her husband comes, usually twice a day, and takes her on a brisk, long walk.

We are beginning to notice changes in Maxine's stature, which we accept as inevitable. But our prayers are that the Lord allow her to walk beside her husband for as long as possible.

Time is always a factor in a nursing facility. While we give 24-hour-day nursing care, we cannot give one-on-one care all that time. How we wish! As Maxine loses more and more control of her body, she requires more time. Like taking more time for bathroom functions, where she cannot be left alone. We do not want to use restraints.

I remember going to see my son and finding him

with wet pants – and sox. How my heart ached to change things! I see this same heartache in Mr. Boggs' face and hear it in his voice when he occasionally finds his "Maxie" wet. He also agonizes over her teeth. "She always took such pride in her pearly white teeth," he tells us. The staff try their best to brush her teeth with morning and bedtime care, but she bites the tooth-brush, holding it between her teeth. If we wait a few seconds, she lets go and you can continue – for a while. Again, time is against us. Mr. Boggs brought in a dental rinse, but her brain dictates that whatever is put into the mouth should be swallowed! The trick now is to use cotton swabs to apply the rinse – without letting her bite the swab.

As I mentioned earlier, when Maxine fed herself, the tendency was **not** to chew and swallow the food before putting more into her mouth. One morning, I remember all too well. At breakfast one of us noticed that she was choking. The aide called for a nurse. I responded and removed two small plastic butter pat tubs from her mouth. It became apparent that she still had something in her throat. Repeated Heimlich maneuvers did not help. Our unit clerk called EMS and I started her on oxygen. Our local hospital treated her and released her just before noon. Diagnosis: Scrapes in the throat from the plastic butter tubs.

Back at the Village she still had a frightened look on her face as she came to lunch. She was eager to eat, but the first bite or two brought trouble. Her lips turned blue and her face a pasty white. We rushed her to her room via wheelchair as I yelled to the unit clerk to call the ambulance back STAT. With her lying on the floor, we tried forward abdominal thrusts. Mr. Boggs was by her head asking the Lord to take care of his "Maxie" and I was desperately praying: "Lord, please don't let me lose her with him standing here watching!" Suddenly, we were able to get an air passage open and started her on oxygen.

Leaving her with an aide and Mr. Boggs, I slipped away a moment to talk to the doctor to explain what we thought the situation was: "She still has something in her throat!"

Back to the hospital they went again, with sirens screaming and Mr. Boggs close behind them. Sure enough, the doctor came from behind the curtain triumphantly holding another little butter tub and saying to Mr. Boggs: "You were right! Here it is! Now she's OK."

While Maxine had a sore throat a few days. she seemed to be "no worse for the wear." But **what a day** for our staff and Mr. Boggs! One we shall never forget.

To prevent a recurrence of such a near-tragedy, new procedures were quickly implemented. Nothing on her tray that was not edible. Have Maxine facing the staff when she was eating. Cut all food into bite-size pieces. Remove the tray and clean the table when she is finished eating.

As time passes, problems change. Maxine no longer feeds herself, but it takes patience to get her to take fluids.

Caring for patients with Alzheimer's disease and related disorders (ADRD) is a real challenge. The plan of care must constantly be adjusted as each individual patient changes. If they are ambulatory, they may be a "wanderer," in which case anything can become a danger to them. It may be that they have forgotten the proper use of every-day articles (which they **may** find when visiting another room). Constant

supervision is a "must" for them. We must continu-
ously re-train and re-instruct our staff in order to meet
the constantly changing needs of our residents.

I consider it a privilege to write this little chapter in
a book I trust will find a wide circulation and helpful
place with many people. While I have concentrated
mostly on one family, be assured that the Boggs'
problems are common to many of our other patients
and to a growing section of our society at large. I hope
you see reflected from these pages the fact that we "on
the inside"' of health care institutions are, after all, just
human beings like all the rest of you, but with our own
mission and niche.

Helps
in
Health Care
Facility
Selection

SELECTING A NURSING CARE FACILITY

What to Look For and Where

by SCOTT R. PUCKETT, C.E.O.
Wesley Manor
Frankfort, Indiana

THE PROCESS OF SELECTING a nursing care facility for a family member or friend will certainly be difficult if you are not prepared. You are entering a field with which most people are unfamiliar, hence they would not know what to look for. To complicate matters, the individuals doing the search are commonly racked with guilt for moving a loved one to a "nursing home." But take heart! This chapter is included in this book to help an inevitable process to go more smoothly for you by giving you some practical "tools" to use in the selection procedure. We hope you will find these things helpful.

It is important to note that even though the media loves to point out nursing homes that neglect/abuse elderly residents, these represent a very small minority. Most facilities these days provide reasonably good care. But if you do your homework, in most localities you can find one of the **excellent** facilities within a reasonable distance.

Alternative Levels/Choices – Assisted Living

One of the first questions to answer is, "What level of care do we need?" Many facilities have what we call "Assisted Living." It may be called by various names in different places, but basically it offers much of the care a nursing home would offer, at about 40 percent to 60 percent of the cost of full nursing home care.

The services offered in these "Assisted Living" wings would include meals, laundry, housekeeping, administered medications, and some organized "activities" or recreation. These people are able to dress themselves and go to the dining room for meals. This kind of care fits the mental/physical condition of **many** older people who mainly need a nurse to see to it that they don't forget to take their medications. Often the medicines are important to the health and well being of a person and must be given on a strict schedule.

Many older people tend to neglect a balanced diet of wholesome food. "Assisted Living" takes care of that, too! So, to repeat, the question is, "What level of care is needed?" No need to pay an average of $80 per day for full nursing care if you can get by with roughly half that much.

Some Observations:

No nursing facility you select is equipped to give a patient **all** they need. It is impossible. A common problem for a nursing home resident is the feeling of isolation. There are social, spiritual and emotional needs we cannot ever fully meet alone. Families must continue to be **as active** as **possible** in the life of the patient.

A Team Effort Is Necessary

Trips, weekends at home, out for lunch, and/or regular visits by **all** family members can make a nursing home stay very positive. It is truly a team effort that is necessary if all the needs of a family member are to be met at this stage of her/his life.

Continue to give them as much power in decision-making as you can. If you, in a rough-shod manner, simply take over everything, one of two things may happen: The family member may become resentful/-suspicious, and make all the rest of the journey a real "pain" for you. Or he/she may become prematurely "fully dependent" and give up altogether. You certainly don't want either of these things to happen. Remember, this person, even though they might have become "like a child" in many ways, still needs to be treated with the dignity and respect you gave them when they were still "in control" of their lives in their own homes. The best rule to go by in any situation is the "Golden Rule" (found in Matthew 7:12).

*   *   *

We now list several things that can help you meet the challenge you face.

1. Identify your family member's specific needs. Tell this to the Social Service Director, Director of Nursing or Administrator. Ask them how well equipped they are to care for your family member's needs.

2. Aim at meeting the Administrator and Director of Nursing. The care you can expect will probably be a direct reflection of their values, experience and commitment to quality. You need to feel very comfortable with these people; they are responsible for the care given in that place.

3. Take a thorough tour of the facility. Stop and speak to an alert resident or two and ask them if they are satisfied with their care.

4. Join them for a meal if possible. How is the food?

5. If the family member can join you on the tour, it would be best.

6. Too often people make decisions based on the lowest daily rate. Remember, you normally get what you pay for. It may be worth paying a few extra dollars a day to get the quality you want. But you should price shop so that you don't end up paying far more than necessary. The average in 1993 was $29,000 a year, or $80 per day.

7. The quality of staff is the most important factor. Are the housekeepers, dietary workers, nurse aides and maintenance people friendly and neat?

8. Ask to see a copy of the facility's two latest State Surveys. Multiple problems here should be a red flag, but it is common for a good facility to have as many as five identified problems to correct. Remember, the Surveyor's job is to find problems, not to praise.

*   *   *

On your "get acquainted" inspection tour of a facility, here are several things that would be well to notice:

A. The obvious –
  - smell of the place;
  - appearance/dress of residents;
  - cleanliness of residents;
  - cleanliness of the facility and rooms;
  - restricted visiting hours (more than the usual 8 a.m. to 8 p.m.);
  - friendliness of the staff – do they smile, say "hello";
  - how active are the residents – what are the activities?
  - the upkeep of the grounds and building;
  - is the place licensed by the state?
  - do they accept Medicare/Medicaid?
  - how far is the facility from your home – or from the residence of the family member who will be visiting most?

B. The not-so-obvious –
  - check their latest few surveys by the State Board of Health;
  - is the facility church-related?
  - is it "for profit" or "not for profit"?
  - how do you feel about the staff you've met?
  - is their staffing ratio at least 3.0 nursing hours/res/day ICF (Intermediate Care Facility)?
  - is their staffing ratio at least 3.3 nursing hours/resident/day SNF (Skilled Nursing Facility)?
  - ask to speak to a Resident Council member;
  - drop by and visit unannounced;
  - are there fire alarms, smoke detectors, sprinklers?
  - is the building design "user friendly" to seniors, i.e., steps?

- are there "support groups" for the family   available?
- is it a "smoke free" facility (including employees)?
- what therapy services are offered to residents?
- are there chapel services or special activities your family member would enjoy?

These are things you should consider **before** committing your loved one to the care of a health care facility. "Settling" in a place is not something you would want to subject someone to very often, or without a strong reason.

Sources of information on nursing facility choices: Your local hospital, doctor, or Council on Aging; or

American Association for Homes of the Aging
Suite 500
901 E Street, N.W.
Washington, D.C. 20004-2037
Phone: 202/783-2242

American Association of Retired Persons
1909 K Street
Washington, D.C. 20049

Alzheimer's Association
Suite 1000
919 N. Michigan Avenue
Chicago, Illinois 60611-9501

I have reserved the last page as a "Rating Chart" for you to fill out after your investigations. I hope you will find it helpful.

Nursing Center Rating System

	Excellent	Good	Average	Fair	Poor
1. Exterior Appearance of Grounds/Buildings	1	2	3	4	5
2. Professionalism of Administrative Staff	1	2	3	4	5
3. Odor	1	2	3	4	5
4. Interior Cleanliness	1	2	3	4	5
5. Appearance of Residents	1	2	3	4	5
6, Visiting Hours	1	2	3	4	5
7. Friendliness & Appearance, Staff	1	2	3	4	5
8. Success of Recent State Surveys	1	2	3	4	5
9. Quality/Quantity of Activities	1	2	3	4	5
10. Quality/Appearance of Meals	1	2	3	4	5
11. Staffing Levels	1	2	3	4	5
12. Location	1	2	3	4	5
13. Facility Layout; Design & Safety	1	2	3	4	5
14. Attractivenes of Resident Rooms	1	2	3	4	5
15. Variety of Services, Chaplain, Beauticians, Therapists	1	2	3	4	5
16. Accept Medicare/Medicaid	1	2	3	4	5
17. Cost of Services Per Day	1	2	3	4	5
18. Staff Turnover in a Year	1	2	3	4	5

Score _____

(18-25 Excellent;

26-33 Very Good: 34-41 Good;

42-49 Average; 50+ Stay Away!)

Caregiving
to
One Family
Typifies
Day-to-Day
Personal Concerns
for
Many
ADRD Patients
Here are helpful "Do's & Don'ts"

CAREGIVER TIPS

May we share with you some **Caregiver Tips** that are good for Alzheimer's Disease and Related Disorders (ADRD)? They work well at home or in Health Care Facilities.

1. Use eye contact. Use care if you must approach from behind so as not to frighten or agitate.
2. Do not speak to them like a child (even if acting like one). Try to keep the communication on an adult to adult level.
3. Do daily tasks the same way each time, and simplify as much as possible, i.e., laying out clothes in the order they should be put on in the morning. Let them help you do simple tasks.
4. At home, use child-proofing kits for cabinets and drawers.
5. Put locks high on doors to discourage wandering out.
6. Go through the house room by room and "Alzheimer Proof." Better to be safe than sorry.
7. Use of touch may be comforting and calming.
8. Communicate calmly. Slow down your speech and actions.
9. Try covers over stove burners that can hide them.
10. If image in mirror frightens, remove or adjust. . . .
11. Use recliners or rockers for wanderers.

12. Be objective. Don't take aggression or other be-
    haviors personally.
13. Strive for consistency. Keep furniture in same
    place.
14. Help patient maintain a connection to the past.
15. Use anything with texture to stimulate sense of
    touch.
16. Do not talk **about** the patient in front of him/her.
17. Call them by name.
18. Give the patient time to hear and respond.
19. Communicate one message at a time.
20. Give praise for simple achievements.
21. Prepare the patient for what is going to happen.
22. Let them do as much as they can for themselves.
23. Don't be afraid to have and use a sense of humor.
24. Look for a reason behind behavior/reactions –
    medication levels, house noises, things outside
    window.
25. Use distractions to redirect.
26. Don't argue facts if they're hallucinating. It's real
    to them!
27. Simplify mealtime – avoid confusion, distraction,
    loud noise, or abrupt movements. Some are over-
    whelmed by a large meal. Try putting one thing
    at a time in front of them. Avoid patterned plates,
    table linens, etc. Encourage to chew, swallow,
    and quietly repeat as needed.
28. Remember: Out of field of vision may be out of mind.
29. Keep this list handy and add to it.

PEACE FOR YOU
AT EVENTIDE

It is an easy thing to compare Dad and Mom's life together to the beauty and splendor of a golden sunset – after a long day filled with sunshine, clouds and a storm or two. The serenity and grace only God can place upon His children's faces is surely seen on the countenance of these two.

Peace has been the strand that kept their ship from being torn apart by the storms of life. It's strong cords ran through the very fibers of our family. Firmly, it held us together as we faced each accident, death and illness that came along. It intertwined it's tranquility within our souls each time Dad and Mom faced turning points in their ministry.

And now, after nine years of dealing with the relentless enemy named "Alzheimer's," that same heaven-sent Peace still gives us strength and courage. Not just endurance. That alone would be great. But eyes to see **disguised blessings** and mercies, right in the "eye" of the storm!

We see God's Spirit at work in the lives of workers and visitors at Grace Village. The unreserved flow of God's love from Dad to Mom, and back again, is plain to all with eyes and a willingness to see.

This boundless love has and will sustain, not only the Boggs family, but each of you through your "troubled waters."

We know our family is only one of a vast multitude

of you chosen to climb "hills of difficulty." We would like to share with you our conviction that the God of all Creation wants to give you each the strength, joy and love our family has long enjoyed. When you're as "rich" as we are in the things of life that really matter, what soul would be so craven as to refrain from sharing a bit of it with others?

As the sun slips softly behind the gloriously colored canvass in the west, for us, it brings tranquility and peace. Why? Because we've always had "the best of both worlds." We have had love, joy and strength for this world, and a bright hope for tomorrow: Eternal Life with Jesus Christ our Lord!

> In His Great Love,
> BARBARA

LOVE IS NOT LOVE
UNTIL IT IS RETURNED?

What did I know of love as just a babe . . .
    Cuddled by precious arms held closely around me?
Selfless and tender was she – the one who held me tight.
    Only a babe. Could I tell her how much I appreciated
    all she was doing for me?
Did I buy her flowers, run to the store, or clean the
      house?
    No. Little ones only receive love.
    They must Learn how to give it.

Mom, you've given us yourself all these years.
    Now it's our turn to give; not receive.
Do we find ourselves loving only when loved in return?
    Talking only to those who can talk back to us?
Now it is our turn to give to you,
    Without expecting anything in return.

You can't respond as once you did.
    But one look into your eyes tells us
How very much you care.
    One glance toward those longing eyes of yours
Unfolds volumes of unspoken warmth.
    It's bottled up within you now, but Praise God,
Heaven will loose your tongue once more
    On that Glorious Day!

I've said all this to remind us that you still want
    To hear the chitter-chatter that goes on
Between husband and wife, mother and children,
    Grandmother and grandchildren, friend and friend.

The need for fellowship lies silent
    Beneath the surface of your being.
It may be hidden, but it is still very much alive!
    Now we must search for new ways
To communicate to you our love
    All the while not giving up on the old ways.

Mom, we know your love for Jesus and for your family
    Has never changed or lessened;
It has only lost its ability to express itself
    As it once did, and expressed it so vivaciously!
Thank you for the love you've given to us, your family!
    The light of it has never dimmed from our hearts
You see – it is within – one need not say a word!

–BARBARA JO MCMUNN
Mother's Day, May 1989

D

Have you ever observed people carrying on emotionally at the funeral of a family member – perhaps abused/neglected parents – saying how great they were and how much they loved them, while you knew the sad facts of the case? The "show" after they were gone did not favorably impress you, did it? "Give me my flowers while I'm alive and can smell them" is another way to put it.

My sister Martha put the idea in yet another beautiful and positive way in her lovely poem, LOVE IS FOR NOW. Thank you, Sister!

LOVE IS FOR NOW

The time to love, my friend, is now,
    Don't wait till you are left alone;
To say how much you thought of those,
    As their departing you bemoan.
On earth their days are numbered well,
    And fleeting moments swiftly fly;
Years have a way of hastening on,
    There is no time to sit and sigh.
Some day your love friends will not need,
    They will have reached their final goal;
For memory's sake do love them now,
    It will enrich and bless your soul.
While promised length of life yet blooms,
    For all, it's threescore years and ten;
In faith I hear your words and deeds,
    "I choose to love you now, my friend."

                   – MARTHA L. SCHAFFER©

THE GREATEST OF THESE

When all things vanish, love remains,
More than emotion's ploy;
Love is a choice made by the will
That gleans devotion's joy.
We must reach forth till we attain
Truth that our Master taught;
The gift of love I must bestow,
Without which all is naught.
This love endures in life's despair,
And hardly sees the wrong;
Its kindness mends a broken heart,
And plants therein a song.

         — MARTHA L. SCHAFFER©

YOU AND I TOGETHER

You and I together, life's hill we've climbed,
Tho' fifty years have come and gone;
The future calls for us to climb on still,
Each step we take — a stepping stone.

Each year that we're together thrills me so,
As every day your love I greet;
To be a part of your life, my heart smiles,
So grateful that our paths did meet.

You and I together, we're still real pals,
And each other's very best friend;
Across the years I've been that special one
To whom you confide at day's end.

This world may be vast, and at times unsure,
But one thing I feel certain of;
As we walk on together hand in hand,
I know I'll always have your love.

         — MARTHA L. SCHAFFER©

THANK YOU, MY FRIEND

Thank you for lending me your faith
     When mine is weak and almost gone;
In heart and soul you've felt my pain,
     I'm grateful for the good you've done.
I need your hope along with faith,
     That I, my duties may fulfill;
And trust, when I, no hope can see,
     To do my best to find God's will.
Your prayers in my behalf I sense,
     They lift me up when I am low;
Your cheerful words light up my path
     To give me courage . . . that will grow.
I thank you for faith, hope and love,
     The kind true friends will surely give;
They radiate within your smile,
     Reflections of the way you live.

– MARTHA L. SCHAFFER©

ADRD

Is

No

Respecter

of

Persons

References

Adamson, D.; Feinauer, L.; Lund, D. and Caserta, M. (1992). Factors affecting marital happiness of caregivers of the elderly in multigenerational families. *American Journal of Family Therapy*, 20(1), 62-70.

Aronson, M. (Ed.) et al (1988). Understanding Alzheimer's Disease: What it is; How to cope with it; Future directions. Overview. Diagnostic. p. 4-11. How to Cope; What do support groups do? p. 191-192. Marks, Jean. Charles Scribner's Sons, New York.

Braitwaite, V. (1992). Caregiving burden: Making the concept scientifically useful and policy relevant. *Research on Aging, 14(1)*, 3-27.

Brody, J. and Cohen, D. (1989). Epidemiologic Aspects of Alzheimer's Disease. *Journal of Aging and Health, 1(*2), 139-149.

Brubaker, T. (Ed.). (1987). *Aging, health, and family: Long-term care.* Newbury Park, CA: Sage.

Cutler, L. (1985, Fall). Counseling caregivers. *Generaerations,* 53-57.

Deimling, G.; Bass, D.; Townsend, A., and Noelker, L. (1989). Care-related stress: A comparison of spouse and adult-child caregivers in shared and separate households. *Journal of Aging and Health, 1*(1), 67-81.

Eisdorfer, C.; Rabins, P. and Reisberg, B. (1991). Alzheimer's disease: Caring for the caregiver. *Patient Care*, November, 109-123.

George, L. and Gwyther L. (1986). Caregiver well-being: A multidimensional examination of family caregivers of demented adults. *Gerontologist, 26*(3), 253-259.

Hay, J. and Ernst, R. (1987). The economic cost of Alzheimer's disease. *American Journal of Public Health, 77*(9), 1169-1175.

Johnson, C. and Catalano, D. (1983). A longitudinal study of family supports to impaired elderly. *Gerontologist, 23*, 612-618.

Kushner, H.S. *When Bad Things Happen to Good People.* Avon Books (1988) Ch. 2, Story of a Man Named Job. Ch. 8, p. 139-140.

Lucado, Max. *The Applause of Heaven.* Word Pub. (1990) p. 5. Moody Bible Institute, *Today in the Word,* p. 37, Oct. 1993.

Moritz, D.; Kasl, S. and Ostfeld, A. (1992). The health impact of living with a cognitively impaired elderly spouse. *Journal of Aging and Health, 4*(2), 244-267.

Ory, M. (1985, Fall). The burden of care. *Generations,* 14-17.

Pallett, P. (1990). A conceptual framework for studying family caregiver burden in Alzheimer's-type dementia. I*MAGE: Journal of Nursing Scholarship, 22*(1),m 52-58.

Peters, G.; Hoyt, D.; Babchuk, N.; Kaiser, M. and Iijma, Y. Primary-group support systems of the aged. *Research on Aging, 9*, 392-416.

Reutter, L. (1984). Family health assessment – an integrated approach. *Journal of Advanced Nursing, 9*, 391-399.

Romeis, J. (1989). Caregiver strain: Toward an enlarged perspective. *Journal of Aging and Health, 1*(2), 188-208.

Seamands, David A. (1985). Healing of Memories. Victor Books. Wheaton, IL. Also: Healing of *Damaged Emotions.* pp. 51-52.

Sommers, T. (1985, Fall). Caregiving: A woman's issue. *Generations,* 9-13.

Tennstedy, S.; Cafferata, G. and Sullivan, L. (1992). Depression among caregivers of impaired elders. *Journal of Aging and Health, 4*(1), 58-76.

Zarit, S. (1985, Fall). New Directions. *Generations,* 6-8.

Zondervan, *The Holy Bible, Amplified Version; The Holy Bible, New International Version.*